The AIDS Bureaucracy

The

AIDS
Bureaucracy

Sandra Panem

HARVARD UNIVERSITY PRESS
Cambridge, Massachusetts
London, England
1988

Library of Congress Cataloging-in-Publication Data

Panem, Sandra, 1946–
  The AIDS bureaucracy / Sandra Panem.
  p. cm.
  Includes index.
  1. AIDS (Disease)—Government policy—United States.   2. AIDS
(Disease—United States—History.   I. Title.
  [DNLM: 1. Centers for Disease Control (U.S.)   2. National
Institutes of Health (U.S.) 3. Acquired Immunodeficiency Syndrome.
4. Delivery of Health Care—organization & administration—United
States.   5. Research—United States.   WD 308 P191a]
RA644.A25P36 1988
362.1'969792—dc19
DNLM/DLC
for Library of Congress   87-22972
                                      CIP
ISBN 0-674-01270-4 (cloth)
ISBN 0-674-01271-2 (paper)

Designed by Gwen Frankfeldt

For my mother, Gertrude Panem,
and in memory of my father, Morris Panem

Acknowledgments

T HE support of many colleagues and friends was indispens-
able in writing this book. Christine Helms, Mary Treuhaft,
Katherine Piva, and Harriet Dorsen offered frequent encourage-
ment and counsel.

I am immeasurably grateful to all of the persons who generously submitted to the interviews and telephone conversations
that allowed me to sort out the events and context of the early
years of the AIDS epidemic. Very special thanks are due to
Edward N. Brandt, Jr.; thanks as well to James Curran, Marcus
Conant, Lawrence Altman, and Maureen Myers. Susan Wool-
len and Diana Coupard provided invaluable assistance in
research and preparation of the manuscript. Susan McGrath,
Laura Walker, and their colleagues in the Brookings Institution
Library have my greatest respect and gratitude.

Many colleagues generously undertook critical readings of
the manuscript. Among them are Christine Helms, Arthur
Silverstein, Walter Bacon, Allen Dyer, Steven Hess, James
Carroll, Dorothy Nelkin, Paul Peterson, and William Check.
Michael Bessie expertly guided me through the publishing
world.

I acknowledge Barbara Sloane for early editorial assistance,
and am grateful to Anita Safran who expertly copyedited the
final text. Howard Boyer has been not only a fine editor, but a
champion of this book.

The AIDS Bureaucracy was written while I was a guest scholar
at the Brookings Institution. I cannot imagine a better place to

have done this work and therefore acknowledge with thanks Bruce MacLaury, Alice Rivlin, and A. Lee Fritschler who supported my guest scholar privileges. I also acknowledge Albert Rees, President of the Alfred P. Sloan Foundation for understanding the distractions of the editorial and publication process.

S.P.

New York
November 1987

Contents

Foreword

I
N THE seven years since AIDS was first recognized in the
United States, remarkable progress has been made in our
understanding of the disease. We know that it is caused by a
particular virus, which is transmitted in sexual intercourse and
in contaminated blood, most frequently passed in syringes
shared by intravenous drug users and from mother to fetus
during pregnancy; it is not transmitted by casual contact or
insect bites. Blood tests for the presence of antibodies to the
AIDS virus, human immunodeficiency virus (HIV), help detect
infection and have almost eliminated transmission through
blood transfusions; the virus itself can be isolated from the
blood and other body fluids. Our knowledge of the epidemiology, natural history, and complications of HIV infection continues to expand and is communicated rapidly in the medical
literature and in frequent conferences. We have strategies for
developing vaccines, antiviral drugs, and therapies for the
complex infections to which AIDS patients are susceptible. One
drug that is directed specifically at the AIDS virus, AZT, already
has been introduced; others are being tested. Models for
organizing care of AIDS patients are being explored. The
international dimensions of the epidemic, particularly its dev-
astating effect in Africa, also have become all too clear.

Sadly, despite these advances, the United States does not
have a plan that would bring the government, academia, and
the private sector into a coordinated effort against AIDS.
Individual units of the government, particularly the Centers for

Disease Control, the National Institutes of Health, and the Food and Drug Administration, have performed superbly notwithstanding the atmosphere of uncertainty, fear, and pressure created by a new and terrifying disease. But no clear strategy of testing and tracking HIV infection has emerged. There is no plan for organizing and financing the care for AIDS patients, no integration of public and private resources for vaccine and drug development, and no overall strategy for public and target-group education. In short, the national response to the most serious epidemic to face the country in decades is primarily the sum of the independent responses of the many components of our health and social services systems.

Why we have failed to develop a coordinated response against AIDS and what we can learn to prepare for future health emergencies is the subject of this book. Dr. Panem does an excellent job of tracing the history of AIDS in the United States, and of describing how the components of our health system interact or fail to interact under both normal and emergency conditions. She presents a thoughtful set of recommendations based on the analysis of the early history of AIDS. Her recommendations will not win everyone's consent, but they represent an attempt to learn from a national tragedy, to deal with immediate deficiencies in our response, and to think about the crisis in generic terms that might improve our response to future medical emergencies. The thoughtful, forward-looking approach of this book makes it an important resource for a more dispassionate debate on how to confront AIDS now and other health crises yet to come.

Samuel O. Thier, M.D.
President, Institute of Medicine
National Academy of Sciences

The AIDS Bureaucracy

AABB	American Association of Blood Banks
ADAMHA	Alcohol, Drug Abuse, and Mental Health Administration
AIDS	Acquired Immune Deficiency Syndrome
AMFAR	American Foundation for AIDS Research
CBO	Congressional Budget Office
CDC	Centers for Disease Control
DOD	Department of Defense
DRR	Division of Research Resources
FDA	Food and Drug Administration
FEMA	Federal Emergency Management Agency
GAO	Government Accounting Office
HCFA	Health Care Finance Administration
HHS	Department of Health and Human Services
HIV	Human Immunodeficiency Virus
HRA	Health Resources Administration
HRSA	Health Resources and Services Administration
HSA	Health Services Administration
HTLV-III	Human T-cell Lymphotropic Virus, type III
IOM	Institute of Medicine
JAMA	*Journal of the American Medical Association*
KSOI	Kaposi's sarcoma and opportunistic infections
LAV	Lymphadenopathy-Associated Virus
MMWR	*Morbidity Mortality Weekly Report*
NCI	National Cancer Institute
NEI	National Eye Institute
NEJM	*New England Journal of Medicine*
NHLBI	National Heart, Lung and Blood Institute
NIAAA	National Institute of Alcohol Abuse and Addiction
NIAID	National Institute of Allergy and Infectious Diseases
NICHHD	National Institute of Child Health and Human Development
NIDA	National Institute of Drug Abuse
NIH	National Institutes of Health
NINCDS	National Institute of Neurological and Communicative Disorders and Stroke
OASH	Office of Assistant Secretary of Health
OMB	Office of Management and Budget
OTA	Office of Technology Assessment
PHS	Public Health Service
SHA	State Health Agency
VA	Veterans Administration

Introduction

History is full of scourges, unpredictable in occurrence and magnitude, which have decimated populations: infectious and often fatal diseases, natural disasters, and the hazards of modern technology. The most recent threat to public health—AIDS, the acquired immune deficiency syndrome—still defies the experience, the biomedical tools, and the institutional structures concerned with the public's health. Six years into the epidemic the head of the World Health Organization stated:

> I don't know of any greater killer than AIDS, not to speak of its psychological, social and economic maiming . . . Everything is getting worse and worse in AIDS and all of us have been underestimating it, and I in particular . . . I thought wait and see—maybe it is not as hot as some are making it appear . . . I definitely admit to a gross underestimate.[1]

In the first five years of the AIDS epidemic scientists achieved stunning successes, such as the rapid identification of the AIDS virus and the development of a diagnostic test. The failures that occurred were of a nonscientific nature: an extraordinarily naive announcement by the government that a vaccine would be developed within two years, and glaring mistakes of judgment that include delaying public information efforts. Examining the reasons for these successes and failures reveals more than an evaluation of how the AIDS epidemic was being handled; it illustrates the difficulties of crafting the appropriate responses to a new disease at the end of the twentieth century.

All epidemics of a new disease can be divided into stages, defined on the basis of information at hand. The initial period always is characterized by unknowns. A second period begins when effective medical treatment or prevention becomes available. A third period, devoted to fine-tuning prevention and intervention, follows. Each stage has problems inherent in it and requires different management approaches. Perhaps the greatest difficulty lies in determining when an epidemic has turned into a "health emergency" that justifies an extraordinary effort.

During the critical initial period, the principal problem is finding the right questions to ask, which requires insightful analysis from the broadest possible perspective. After the right questions are framed, the organization of an effective response is still complicated by a number of things. First, preliminary research must be done to confirm that the questions are indeed the right ones before a focused research program can be mounted. Second, no one person and no one part of the health establishment directs the effort. Third, there is the complex matter of reallocating resources from already existing research programs. And finally, the response is often limited by lack of ideas (because the problem is too new to have stimulated them) and by a shortage of available professional personnel.

In contrast, research done in the second period, after the disease is better defined, benefits from strategies used to manage research in other established fields of biomedical science. These strategies first entail the enumeration and ordering of known, but unproved avenues of investigation; the number of these avenues that can be explored will be determined by the level of available resources. And regardless of the research advances, health and social services, as well as public education, must be provided during each stage of the epidemic.

In the AIDS epidemic, the division between the initial and second period occurred when the virus that causes AIDS was identified and accepted. Researchers could then abandon less fruitful lines of investigation and use the newly discovered virus as a tool for preventing spread of the disease—for example, by developing methods of testing blood for antibodies to the AIDS virus. As a first major benefit, this made it possible to ensure the safety of the national blood supply. Scientists began then to look for drugs that would inhibit viral infection and considered the development of a vaccine against AIDS. Transition from the first to the second stage occurred between fall 1983 and spring 1984.

The third stage of the AIDS epidemic will occur when effective treatment for AIDS is developed. Then research and patient care will focus on how they can be improved. When will the third stage begin? Research is unpredictable and there is no way to predict exactly when effective treatments will be discovered. This fact alone forces attention to the major failures in managing the AIDS epidemic—too little attention to public education for disease prevention, and not enough strategic planning for providing health and social services.

In formal public health terms, an epidemic occurs with one or more unanticipated cases of disease. But no public policy guidelines exist for determining when an epidemic becomes an emergency nor for activating an emergency management plan. Although the decision to declare a health emergency may appear to require only straightforward technical analysis, it involves complex social value judgments and sensitivity to public fears.

It is not clear when AIDS should have been recognized as requiring an extraordinary response—both by researchers and by the purveyors of health care services. After how many cases? How many deaths? How broad a geographic distribution? Did AIDS become a serious problem only after it was featured in national newspapers and on the nightly news? After it was seen to affect both hetero- and homosexuals?

The AIDS emergency makes a compelling case study of the public health services' capability because of the unprecedented dimension of the crisis. The thesis of this book is that the extreme nature of AIDS so stresses the system that cracks appear that are ordinarily obscured. For example, when the crisis surfaced, there was no clear-cut division of responsibilities among local, state, and federal officials for health, education and social service delivery. The decision makers at the national, state, and local levels were trapped in the prerogatives of office and influenced by suspicion, personal ambition, rivalries, societal and political sensibilities, all intensified by the distorting glare of publicity.

I aim to identify factors that can lead to the most effective and timely response to future novel health emergencies; I do not intend this to be a definitive history of the AIDS epidemic. The events of the first five years—from the detection of early signs of a new disease in late 1979 to the acceptance of a virus as the cause of AIDS in the spring of 1984—suffice to expose the problems of responding to a new disease. The discovery of the AIDS virus clearly demarcates the end of the initial period of the epidemic, an appropriate place to end this case study. Whatever happens as the AIDS epidemic expands and the disease is viewed as a long-term and perhaps chronic health problem, analysis of the first few years remains timely because of its relevance for future crisis management.

This book centers on the AIDS bureaucracy—the institutions on which we must rely during a health emergency. Particular attention is paid to the Public Health Service (PHS), especially the National Institutes of Health (NIH) and the Centers for Disease Control (CDC). I concentrate on these two PHS agencies because their activities formed the majority of federal AIDS efforts in the initial stages of the epidemic. Less attention is paid to the Food and Drug Administration (FDA), whose activities became really notable only after the AIDS virus was identified, because methods of detecting viral infection and tests for antiviral drugs could not be developed until then. Moreover, because development of patient care strategies and health service delivery lagged behind research and epidemiology (one of the problems in the management of AIDS), analysis of specific programs directed at patient care receives less attention than the activities of CDC and NIH.

The discussion of the various agencies shows how the lack of communication within and among the various groups exacerbated the effort to manage the AIDS epidemic. The biomedical research establishment, for instance, was criticized for slowness in its response to the crisis and for reliance on a peer review system whose incentives may encourage personal ambition at the expense of the overall scientific effort. The dynamics of the system and its components become clearer when examined in the light of the history of our health institutions. Thus I briefly trace the evolution of public health and research agencies since the 1700s.

Money is a crucial factor in the AIDS effort. Hence I take a close look at the federal budget process to show the vital role politics plays in determining fiscal priorities and to assess the influence of advocacy groups in obtaining funds for special projects. The conflict between the need for technical information and the desire to protect trade secrets is also examined. Just as this book is not the definitive chronicle of the AIDS epidemic, it is not an exhaustive analysis of the development of health institutions or the political process of setting the federal budget. Rather, my intention is to make the reader aware of the institutional and political context in which to view the initial period of the AIDS epidemic. The argument draws heavily on secondary sources of information; the important scholarly literature on health planning, budget and organization analysis, and public administration is not directly treated in this book.

Following the examination of the institutional and political milieu, I discuss the public relations and communications aspects of the AIDS crisis—particularly how the media affected public perceptions and misconceptions about the disease; the problems caused by the lack of channels of communication with those at high risk for AIDS; and how the media contributed to politicization of the crisis, thus exacerbating it. The book concludes with suggestions of ways to improve the management of future novel health emergencies. I explore public policy options that might facilitate crisis management by forcing attention to problems one would easier deny.

AIDS is clearly the most important public health problem of current times because of its deadliness, the hidden nature of infection at a time when the virus can be spread, and the daunting projections of the human and economic toll that will occur without scientific, medical, and social policy advances. AIDS also challenges society to treat the disease as a health problem, even if social mores must be confronted. Finding the effective treatment for AIDS is the goal of all; finding a way to respond quickly and effectively to a new health emergency is the goal to which this book may contribute.

1

The Advent of AIDS

IN LATE 1979, physicians at university medical centers began to hear anecdotal reports of cases of Kaposi's sarcoma (KS)—a rare skin cancer usually found in older men of Mediterranean origin—appearing in previously healthy young homosexual men. These shared reports took about a year to arouse concern. Dr. Alvin Friedman-Kien, a professor of dermatology at New York University who was among the first to recognize AIDS as a new clinical entity, recalled:

> An internist I know called me up and said he had a very unusual case . . . I looked at the lesions [brown spots on the patient's legs] and said this looks like Kaposi's sarcoma. I couldn't believe I was seeing that in a young man. It is a rare disease—about 1 to 2 cases occurring in every 600,000 cases . . . What we were looking at in 1981 was a new disease that had never occurred before in an epidemic form or in the number and severity we were seeing it.[1]

On June 5, 1981, the Centers for Disease Control (CDC) reported the appearance of pneumonia in five young men during the previous six months. Five cases of pneumonia in eight months at a major medical center is hardly notable. Yet suspicion was aroused because the patients shared several characteristics: they were young, their pneumonias were caused by *Pneumocystis carinii*, a type of infection generally seen only in patients who were severely immunosuppressed because of the chemotherapy used to treat a known disease (factors absent from these patients' histories), and all five were homosexuals.

A few months earlier, some cases of Kaposi's sarcoma (KS) and opportunistic infections (infections ordinarily checked by the body's own defenses) had caught the attention of Dr. William Foege, director of the CDC, who discussed them with Dr. Edward N. Brandt, Jr., assistant secretary for health in the Department of Health and Human Services. Brandt subsequently recalled that the reports of these KSOI cases first seemed to him to be a clustered reaction to an unidentified drug.

One month later, in a July 4, 1981, report of the CDC, a group led by Friedman-Kien described KS in twenty homosexual men in New York and six homosexual men in California. Some of these patients also had *Pneumocystis carinii* pneumonia and other infections of a type previously seen in patients receiving immunosuppressive drugs. The CDC report concluded that such an occurrence was highly unusual, and it urged physicians to be on the lookout for it in homosexual men. At about the same time, KSOI was recognized in some male drug addicts in New York and California who denied engaging in homosexual activities (see Table 1).

Reinforcing the first signals were requests the CDC received in late 1980 and early 1981 for dispensing pentamidine—a drug used for treatment of pneumocystis pneumonia in patients whose underlying cause of illness was unknown. Pentamidine was then an infrequently used "orphan" drug that could only be obtained through a physician's request to the CDC.

Orphan drugs are those used to treat conditions that occur too infrequently to allow a drug manufacturer to produce them at a profit. The government encourages manufacture of such drugs in a number of ways. In 1981, CDC acted as a guaranteed market for pentamidine, which it then dispensed. In that year the unusual number of requests for the drug, together with the reports of the CDC's *Morbidity and Mortality Weekly Report* (*MMWR*), led Dr. Foege to appoint a task force, headed by Dr. James Curran, to look into the matter.

Jim Curran, an energetic and outspoken public health officer, had trained in the CDC's Epidemiological Intelligence Service. He had specific experience in tracking sexually transmitted

Table 1.   The Initial Stage of the AIDS Epidemic:
            Late 1979–Spring 1984

Early Signs

1979–1980   Anecdotal reports of Kaposi's sarcoma in young, homo-
            sexual men in New York City, San Francisco and Los
            Angeles

1981   Report on 5 cases of *Pneumocystis carinii* pneumonia in
                homosexual men in *MMWR*
            Increased requests for pentamidine
            PHS AIDS task force formed
            NCI meeting on Kaposi's sarcoma
            Reports on KSOI in the peer reviewed medical literature

            The Emergence of Risk Groups

1982   Hypothesis that "poppers" cause KSOI discounted
            KSOI diagnosed in Haitians in the United States
            AIDS defined as a syndrome
            Transfusion-related AIDS reported
            Pediatric AIDS reported

            The Hunt for the Cause of AIDS

1983   Immunodeficiency in female sexual partners of men with
                AIDS reported
            Hypothesis that AIDS is caused by a retrovirus is proposed
            Recommendations for preventing the spread of AIDS are
                published in *MMWR*
            GAO audits NIH and CDC AIDS activities
            Science publishes article on LAV by Montagnier and
                colleagues
            Congressional hearings in Washington on the "Federal
                Response to AIDS"
            Committee on Government Operations issues report on
                "Federal Response to AIDS" with dissenting views
            French scientists file first U.S. patent application

1984   Robert Gallo's group reports growth of HTLV-3 *in vitro*
            Margaret Heckler announces discovery of HTLV-3 as the
                cause of AIDS
            First HHS patent filed
            Independent isolation of an AIDS retrovirus, ARV, re-
                ported by Levy and colleagues

diseases—the late 1970s name for venereal disease. When he accepted his new assignment in the spring of 1981, no one could have predicted what Curran has since and frequently said: "Some of us will devote our careers to this disease." Nor could he have foreseen the on-the-job training as an epidemiologic diplomat, scientific counsellor, and media personality that the growing concern about AIDS would offer him.

In less than four years the five-man task force, initially known as the Task Force on Kaposi's Sarcoma and Opportunistic Infections, was to grow into the AIDS Activity in the Center for Infectious Diseases. In fiscal 1985, the AIDS Activity alone had a staff of eighty and a budget of approximately $10 million, and that represented only part of the CDC's AIDS effort that year.[2]

Between August 1981 and May 1982 the *MMWR* published no new information about the developing epidemic, but the efforts to understand it grew apace. In September 1981 the National Cancer Institute (NCI), recognizing a public health crisis as well as a scientific opportunity to learn about cancer and opportunistic infections, organized a workshop in Bethesda, Maryland, to which fifty-four scientists and physicians of diverse interests and backgrounds were invited. According to Arthur Levine,[3] who headed these initiatives, the NCI took the lead because the presenting symptom was often a cancer (KS), and because the institute had "spare pocket change." Among the results of the workshop was the recognition that the syndrome was not an epidemic of cancer, as originally feared, but an illness that put its victims at risk for developing KS as well as numerous opportunistic infections: a cancer epidemic was thus the first of many hypotheses to be tested and discarded. By the time the first reports about patients with KSOI appeared in the peer-reviewed medical literature in December 1981, a consensus was forming among scientists who had been following the phenomenon for over a year that it was a new and unique disease syndrome.[4] Further, the leading hypothesis was that a single unknown event—perhaps infection—would be found responsible for the immunodeficiency observed in these patients.

As interest in the disease broadened, another group of

patients was identified. These were healthy homosexual men who displayed persistent lymphadenopathy, which is often an indication that something is causing the immune system to fight off an infection, raising the possibility that lymphadenopathy was an early indication of developing KSOI. Curran and other CDC epidemiologists became convinced that they were observing the tip of an iceberg that concealed unanswered questions and problems, including other possible manifestations of this disease. As the doctors toured the country to speak about the problem, they began to use the iceberg image as a visual device to emphasize their concerns.

The detailed collection of patients' medical and social histories assembled by the CDC, which maintains a staff of trained medical investigative reporters in its Epidemiological Intelligence Service (EIS) for just this purpose, is one of the most powerful tools for tracking disease. By early 1982 EIS officers had defined two groups of KSOI patients. In one group were homosexual men, many of whom had had many sexual partners. A good proportion of these men used "poppers"—recreational drugs (amyl and butyl nitrate) that enhance sexual pleasure. The second group at risk was composed of heterosexual, bisexual, and homosexual men who were abusers of intravenously injected drugs. Social mores among such drug abusers encourage the sharing of hypodermic needles, so that this group was long known to suffer from the spread of blood-borne infectious diseases, such as that caused by hepatitis B virus.

As the body of information about the patients and the manifestations of the disease grew, more hypotheses were suggested: an infectious agent was being transmitted sexually; the infectious agent was being transmitted by direct blood contact; unidentified factor(s) associated with homosexual behavior might cause or allow the expression of an immune defect; and substances such as poppers might be responsible for the syndrome. Since none of the social factors—promiscuity, drugs, other habits—could be linked to *all* the patients, the odds seemed to be that KSOI was a contagious disease.

By the spring of 1982 approximately two hundred such cases had been detected, and the number was doubling every six months. Moreover, the disease was occurring in clusters, which reinforced the hypothesis that an infectious agent was at work. In addition, KSOI cases included a few women and some bisexual men, indicating that gender or sexual preference did not determine susceptibility to disease. Furthermore, a number of cases were detected in Haitians who had recently come to the United States. And in July 1982 KSOI was reported in three patients with hemophilia A.[5] The cases of hemophilia confirmed the original tentative conclusion of the epidemiologists that this was an infectious disease.

As epidemiologic information grew, the pattern of transmission of KSOI was found to mimic closely the spread of hepatitis B virus, which is transmitted sexually and through contact with contaminated blood and bodily fluids. This pattern, coupled with the knowledge that many viruses show preference for infecting lymphocytes, and that some viral infections induce immunosuppression, strengthened the prevailing hypothesis that KSOI would be due to a blood-borne virus. That hypothesis gained credibility with the identification of contaminated blood transfusions as a means of spreading the disease. Because patients with hemophilia A most frequently lack a clotting protein known as Factor VIII, they were treated with doses of Factor VIII extracted from large pools of human blood. In the United States, the blood was obtained via voluntary blood donations at not-for-profit blood banks or at plasma collection facilities. Therefore, patients who received blood concentrates containing Factor VIII were potentially exposed to blood from hundreds of individuals. In contrast, blood used for transfusions in hospital settings came from individual donors. Yet in the cases of AIDS among hemophiliacs and transfusion recipients who did not belong to other high-risk groups, careful medical detective work uncovered a pattern: these AIDS patients had received blood from some donors who had later developed AIDS.

Throughout the summer of 1982, scientists across the country were involved in experiments designed to increase their under-standing of KSOI. By September of that year the uniqueness of the disease was clear, and the CDC, which recognized 593 cases with a 41 percent mortality rate,[6] gave it a name: "This group of clinical entities, along with its specific immune deficiency, is now called acquired immune deficiency syndrome (AIDS)."[7]

Although the disease was now named, it was not close to being understood. Was AIDS a single syndrome with a common cause or was it a series of diseases? Was there a single viral agent? What kind of virus would it be? If AIDS was caused by an infectious virus, was it likely to be easily spread and what were the populations at risk for developing disease?

Answers to these questions would be essential for establish-ing basic research priorities and appropriate public health policies. For example, if the etiologic agent was not a virus, AIDS might be susceptible to some forms of antibacterial or antifungal drug therapy. If the cause of disease was viral, knowing the nature of the virus was imperative, for antiviral drug therapy in the early 1980s was available for only a very few viral infections. A viral disease might be fought by way of developing a successful vaccine. But even though preventive vaccination against viral disease has a 200-year history, some viral diseases—such as the common cold—are not amenable to vaccination. The most important thing was to pinpoint the routes of disease transmission. Even in the absence of definitive treatment and failure to determine the causative agent, once the spread of disease was understood then strategies of public education could be developed to prevent exposure. Public health officials were just beginning to formulate the problems. As then Assistant Secretary of Health Edward Brandt recalled,

Frankly we did not realize how complex the disease was until mid-1982 . . . Up until then most of us were pretty well convinced that we had a relatively straightforward infectious disease and that basi-cally, if we could find the agent, it would just be a matter of writing the prescription and the problem would be solved. Boy, was that wrong. That was dead wrong. It turned out to be much, much more complicated than anything we had ever dreamed of.[8]

As a public health emergency AIDS most closely resembles the polio epidemics of the 1940s and 1950s, notably in the public panic that accompanied both, their viral etiology, the attention paid to both by the media, and the fact that when each disease appeared in epidemic proportions, neither preventive nor effective treatments were available. Another similarity is the role of a popular figure in mobilizing public support for research: President Roosevelt's paralysis as a result of polio and Rock Hudson's fight with AIDS in the mid-1980s. Although these parallels are strong, one difference is crucial: there was little early sympathy for victims of AIDS because those initially at high risk—homosexual men, Haitian immigrants, and drug addicts—were not in the mainstream of society. In contrast, sympathy for polio patients was extensive, especially because those at highest risk were children. Polio elicited such an outpouring of sympathy that the first modern nationwide attempt to raise money for a medical research campaign—the Mothers March of Dimes organized by the National Foundation for Infantile Paralysis—was a remarkable success.

Media coverage of AIDS increased as the problem began to affect the blood supply and as the numbers of AIDS cases grew. In May 1983 two articles in the *Journal of the American Medical Association (JAMA)* were on AIDS in pediatric patients. The parents of all the child victims were members of groups at high risk for the disease. In one article Dr. James Oleske and colleagues reported the syndrome in eight children and concluded that "children living in high-risk households are susceptible to AIDS and that sexual contact, drug abuse, or exposure to blood products is not necessary for disease transmission." The second article, by a group led by Dr. Arye Rubinstein, said: "We speculate that a perinatal or in utero transmission of EBV [a virus] can induce an infectious immunodeficiency." In the companion editorial, Dr. Anthony Fauci, from the National Institutes of Allergy and Infectious Diseases in Bethesda, analyzed these reports, speculating on the possible casual transmission of AIDS in the household settings.[9] The media picked up these stories, raising a great public alarm: fear then neutralized sympathy, even for the children. For the findings brought up a possibility that this incurable and lethal disease might spread by casual contact, thereby putting untold numbers of people at risk.

Read carefully, the *JAMA* articles and editorial contain many caveats against any likelihood of such casual transmission. Yet the popular interpretation of the *JAMA* news turned a mere possibility into a near certainty. And Fauci, a meticulous scientist who had chosen his words for a medical audience, became an object of the homosexual community's ire, accused of singlehandedly turning its members—and particularly AIDS patients—into lepers overnight.[10] So, not for the first or last time, passions erupted as a result of misunderstanding and simplifications that led to distortions. These in turn contributed to the perception some members of the gay community had of official insensitivity to its problems.[11]

May 1983 produced further surprises. Two articles in *Science* magazine targeted as a possible AIDS agent members of the group of viruses known as retroviruses. This startling news was followed by a press conference at which Assistant Secretary Brandt labeled AIDS the number one health priority. It was also the first time that Brandt had spoken publicly about AIDS. Looking back at his statement and its timing, he explains:

I consider naming AIDS the number one public health priority to be a symbolic declaration, but also to emphasize to the people working on the problem that in fact they were working on something important to man, that everything else was going to take a back seat, and we were going to sacrifice, if necessary, other efforts to accomplish this major goal . . . Somehow we weren't getting that message across, and by that time [spring 1983] I came to figure out that in Washington, you have to have a short phrase to get anybody's attention. Calling it the number one health priority in the country was something that everyone would listen to. It is also something that would get in the media.[12]

Brandt, appointed in 1981[13] as assistant secretary for health and head of the PHS, was charged with leading the federal AIDS effort. In that capacity he had to represent the administration's position and serve as a lightning rod for the criticism directed at that position. Yet even ardent critics of the federal AIDs effort gave him good marks. In the April 1985 *Mother Jones*, Ginny Apuzzo, of the National Gay Task Force, said of Brandt, "I will stand by my criticisms of him . . . but I think fundamentally we are dealing with a man of integrity and competence who came to care a great deal about this issue."[14] Brandt succeeded in opening and maintaining a dialogue between the nonconformist homosexual community and a conservative, often hostile administration. That the AIDS issue was not more politicized during his four years at HHS credits an objective approach to his public health mandate.

A Tale of Two Cities

The two cities in which AIDS first appeared—New York and San Francisco—differed dramatically in the groups at risk, the resources available, and the local political responses. The difference in the course of action may be attributed to the fact that San Francisco's political spectrum included a prominent and active homosexual community, whereas the New York group was made up of isolated constituencies with no community standing or clout.

In San Francisco, a city of 716,000 people, over 95 percent of AIDS cases in 1985 were among homosexual men.[15] By the summer of that year 1,308 AIDS cases were reported: 12 percent of all the cases in the United States. Health officials estimated that over a quarter of the city's entire male population was at high risk for developing AIDS, and that 1 in 700 had clinical AIDS. As early as 1981 the country health department established a task force to deal with the syndrome, and in 1983 San Francisco General Hospital, the major public hospital, devoted a unit to the exclusive treatment of AIDS patients. Other local efforts included joint community–public health programs to provide psychological and social assistance and to distribute educational materials.

In New York, a city of 7.16 million, 33 percent of the nation's

AIDS cases, or 3,757 cases, were reported by the summer of 1985. The estimate for the number of males in New York City infected with the AIDS virus at that time was 1 in 400 (0.25 percent). Approximately 30 percent of these men were not homosexuals but intravenous drug abusers or recent Haitian arrivals. Despite these numbers, in a city that frequently has a hospital bed occupancy rate of over 90 percent, exclusive use of a public facility for AIDS treatment was not yet officially considered.[16]

The differences in approach by the two cities included news coverage. As early as 1982 the San Francisco papers ran daily stories about the epidemic. In contrast, with the exception of the *New York Native,* other papers serving the homosexual community, and occasionally the *Village Voice,* New York news-papers were silent about AIDS. The establishment East Coast press has been accused of avoiding coverage of the initial period of the epidemic because it perceived AIDS as a "gay disease."[17] Yet even with increased reporting the criticism persisted. For example, in spring 1985 the *New York Times* was criticized for continuing to handle AIDS only as a medical science story and failing to voice the concerns of those who were most affected. Numerous explanations have been suggested for why the East Coast press lagged behind the West Coast press in covering all aspects of the AIDS epidemic (see discussion in Chapter 9), but the general lack of coverage in the early years of the epidemic is well documented.

In one analysis of New York City's response to AIDS, Dennis Altman, an Australian political scientist, contrasted New York's attitude with that of San Francisco:

Why has New York failed? Perhaps the most striking thing about San Francisco's response is that Mayor Dianne Feinstein has made AIDS a priority and publicly stressed this frequently in ways that affect the whole city bureaucracy. No senior official in San Francisco could say, as one is reported to have said here, that he is not sure this is a crisis—or even an epidemic. San Francisco had responded to AIDS as a public health crisis, not merely the issue of one community.[18]

The two chief public health officials of the two cities had different professional priorities and personal styles. In the early 1980s Dr. Mervyn Silverman was a gregarious man in his late forties. He had moved to San Francisco from Witchita, Kansas, where he ran the public health department in the mid-1970s. When AIDS struck San Francisco in 1981, Silverman had been director in its department of public health for four years. He enjoyed the reputation of a competent and dedicated professional, and often appeared on local San Francisco TV talk shows. In his assessment of AIDS at the time, the major problem was effective public education.

In contrast to Silverman's mercurial animation was the demeanor of New York City's commissioner of public health. Dr. David J. Sencer came to New York City in 1982 after a brief sojourn in the pharmaceutical industry. From 1960 to 1977 he had been at the CDC, rising to become the agency's director. In an unkind turn of fate, Sencer's stewardship coincided with a crash vaccination program to combat the swine flu, an epidemic that never materialized. He took the public and political heat for the public's displeasure. Although seen as a real public health hero by some students of public health emergency management, Sencer's subsequent low-key demeanor in New York clearly showed the battle scars. And whereas Silverman's conversations on AIDS were charged with energy and optimism, Sencer's comments reflected the experiences of over twenty-five years as a public health professional as well as an appreciation for the complexities of the problems, the limitations of resources and political options, and the knowledge that, once again, he had become a target of public criticism and contention. Sencer considered housing for IV drug addicts and AIDS patients as his major problem regarding AIDS. Despite their differences, the two men shared a genuine commitment to dealing with the problems specific to each city in a way that would most benefit public health.

In both cities measures to fight AIDS became the focus of civil liberties issues, reflecting the skepticism of the homosexual community that the establishment would respect their civil rights. But even here, the focus differed. In New York the most vocal civil liberties debate initially seemed to center on patient confidentiality in the screening of blood. In San Francisco, the most prominent public debate crystallized around the closing of bath houses and the right of the government to police sexual activity for reasons of public health. In other cities—Miami, New Orleans, Boston, and Chicago—the plot was the same but the script was written in the regional vernacular.

The Bath House Fracas

From the very beginning of the epidemic, one thing was consistent about AIDS—the disease was spread during sexual activity between homosexual men. Anything that increased the chances of exchanging semen and blood increased the risk of contracting the disease. In San Francisco, bath houses had flourished during the 1970s as places where homosexual men could gather and engage in frequent and often anonymous sex. As the epidemiology of AIDS evolved, restrictions on sexual activity seemed the most effective way to limit the spread of the disease. The bath houses became the focus of a fierce debate, with some arguing in favor of the government's closing them and others arguing for voluntary self-policing and using the bath houses as the site of a public education campaign. Public Health Director Mervyn Silverman reflects in retrospect on his side of the story:

[About late 1982] the Mayor wanted the bath houses closed, and I wanted the bath houses closed because they obviously . . . were where AIDS was being spread. . . This is basically a behavioral disease, because if you don't practice certain behavior, you're not going to get the disease. Now if I'm going to change behavior, I have to do it as a protective measure, not as a policeman. You don't get people to change behavior too much as a cop. So I decided to educate across the community . . . In April 1983, the rectal gonorrhea [a common venerally spread disease among gay men] rate in San Francisco had dropped 75 percent [indicating that education and fear] obviously had had its impact. I also realized that in trying to balance

this issue, that [concerning sex] whether it's homosexual or heterosexual, you have pretty much a bell shaped curve. People at one end
who are celibate, or monogamous, and it's not an issue. You have
people on the other end who would crawl across glass to have a sexual
encounter. And in between [there are people who with education
change their behavior] . . . That's what I think happened. The
attendance at bath houses went down and some closed.

But in April 1983 the attendance at bath houses seemed to be
increasing. Silverman attempted to get the homosexual community to request that the bath houses be closed. Unsuccessful
in mobilizing grassroots action, he "decided to go for regulations and said, 'Okay, you want to stay open as a bath
house/sex club, fine. But you can't do certain things.' [Well, the
politics of City Hall didn't allow] that to happen. Hearings were
going to be held; they were postponed . . . It was getting close
to the 1984 Democratic National Convention . . . the hearings
were cancelled . . . Then, the November elections were coming
up, and nobody would get near it [the issue] with a ten-foot
pole."

After several months of stormy discussions and temporary
restraining orders issued by the courts, a compromise solution
to the bath house issue was found.

Now the bath houses are supposed to police themselves, and we
will send people in to see that it's done. Undercover—I don't know
how you go undercover when you're naked, but anyway, we will
monitor these establishments. But . . . you can't police safe sex; you
can only police no sex . . . Looking back at the bath house issue, the
Mayor [Feinstein] has said if this had been a heterosexual disease, I
would have closed the bath houses immediately. And she's right,
because it wouldn't have been a bath house; it would have been a
whore house—it would have been a girlie show or some porno film—
you close it, that has no impact. Who is going to rise up? Who is going
to be concerned in the straight community because you close the
whore house? With AIDS, we were trying to look at the community
as the patient. But very few people think in terms of public health.
They think in terms of medicine. I had to make sure that I didn't
turn the patients off, but to try to turn them on to what I was trying
to say.[19]

The difficulties in resolving the bath house issue thus stemmed from confusion of scientific with political concerns, and multiple definitions of the issue. The director of public health, whose credibility derived from medical knowledge, was unwilling to act, on the basis of his political judgment that closing the bath houses would disrupt efforts to limit the spread of the disease through effective public education. The mayor seemed unwilling to act politically when the initiative did not come from the person charged with speaking for the scientific community. Vocal gay activists, such as some members of the San Francisco AIDS Foundation, would not call for bath houses closing because they defined the problem first as a civil liberties question (that is, infringement of the right to assembly and sexual freedom), and only second as a public health or education issue.

In January 1985, three months after he closed the bath houses, Silverman resigned. Rumors circulated in San Francisco that his resignation was related not only to the bath house fracas, but to broader questions of the relationship between the mayor's office and the department of public health.[20]

Protecting the Blood Supply

The central problem in developing a new policy to protect the nation's blood supply was to decide when the evolving body of information had become convincing enough to justify disrupting an established system. The problem arose because the facts about how dangerous a risk AIDS presented were continuously changing. The problem was further complicated by the way in which the blood supply is controlled.

The national blood policy represents a pluralistic, private-sector approach to planning rather than a central, federal government-directed approach, despite the regulation of the manufacture and use of blood products by the Food and Drug Administration. The privately run American Blood Commission implements the "lion's share" of the national blood policy. Although partially funded by the federal government, the commission has no enforcement power or statutory mandate to facilitate oversight of the national blood supply.[21]

Before the discovery of the AIDS virus and the subsequent development of sensitive laboratory tests to detect the antibody to the virus, there was no reliable way to tell whether a person had been infected by the agent of this new disease: the length of time elapsed between infection and the appearance of clinical symptoms was unknown. The problem for those managing the U.S. blood supply was how to minimize the chance of using contaminated blood by screening for high-risk donors.

In the absence of a laboratory tool, the most promising means of identifying individuals at high risk was examining a potential donor's behavioral history, specifically sexual practices and use of IV drugs. But such activities were not readily admitted because they carried social stigmas and were often susceptible to criminal penalty. The socially responsible act of donating blood would have as counterpoint admitting to behavior that might be punishable; and the need to screen out contaminated blood was juxtaposed with the need to maintain sufficient levels of blood for medical purposes. In 1980 voluntary donors provided almost 98 percent of the more than 11 million units of whole blood collected in the United States.[22] A significant percent of this blood was donated by men, often single, between twenty-five and forty-five years of age, and blood bankers were afraid that the loss of these donations could compromise the adequacy of the blood supply. In the absence of blood tests, the situation called for guidelines for voluntary donor deferral.

Throughout early 1983 information concerning the transmission of AIDS through blood transfusion and blood products increased, but the word was not always reaching responsible health officials. As quoted in Fettner and Check's book *Truth About AIDS,* Joseph Bove, representing the American Association of Blood Banks at the CDC's December 1982 meeting to discuss the guidelines for donor deferral, reacted to suggestions that this step be taken by questioning in disbelief: "[Do] we want to take all these sweeping measures just because one baby got AIDS after transfusion from a person who later came down with AIDS—and there may be a few other cases."[23] Bove's skepticism toward official pronouncements was a result of a dearth of information. To implement a policy change he needed to be convinced by more than what seemed to be isolated instances of blood contamination.

Dr. Jay Menitove, a blood banking official in Wisconsin who served on several AIDS task forces, confirmed that some of the early attempts by CDC to alert the blood banks were met with skepticism. Menitove speculated that the skepticism might in part be attributed to the informal channels the CDC sometimes used to convey information to blood bank officials, such as phone conversations.[24] Thus the type of information and the way in which it was transmitted may have contributed to slow acceptance of the problem.

The answer to one question raised by AIDS in hemophilia patients—How widely contaminated were some blood products?—was to be answered less than two years after that December 1982 meeting, when it was reported that virtually every patient with hemophilia in North America and Europe who had utilized Factor VIII (an extract from pooled plasma) manufactured in the United States showed evidence of exposure to the virus that causes AIDS. But even before a test to detect the particular virus that causes AIDS was developed, careful record keeping and epidemiology had pointed to an infectious agent present in some blood products. That epidemiologic information was collected by the CDC. At the August 1983 congressional hearings, Bove testified that he had learned only that morning that the CDC was regularly supplying information to the national Hemophilia Foundation: "But the three major blood collecting organizations have not received that information. Now that I have learned that it is available, I will see if I can get it; but why did I have to learn it here this morning in this way?"[25]

Bove's frustration—both in late 1982 and again in August 1983—raises questions about the most effective way of exchanging and acting on information. The presumption is that it is the federal government's job to disseminate information. Yet the professional recipient of the information bears some responsibility for taking the information seriously.

The skepticism of the blood banking community about the real risk that AIDS presented, the concern of the homosexual community that the growing public fear of AIDS would result in a discriminatory backlash against them, and the anxiety expressed by the Hemophilia Foundation and others created an acrimonious atmosphere in which to develop policy. Considering the emotional tenor of debate, the divergent opinions were remarkably quickly melded into a national consensus on blood donation policy. However, public confusion remained a problem in developing the guidelines because of misconceptions over the point in the blood donation process at which AIDS might be transmitted. Many believed wrongly that the disease could be contracted by a donor during the act of donating blood. The guidelines developed in early 1983 by a PHS task force were published in March 1983 in the *MMWR*, as detailed recommendations calling for voluntary deferral of blood donations by members of high-risk groups.[26] At that time the high-risk groups were still defined as homosexual men, IV drug abusers, and recent Haitian entrants to the United States.

Not all health policy changes derive from scientific evaluation of data; politics may also play a role, as was clear in the bath house controversy. Early in January 1983 some members of the political right wing, who had introduced legislation in Texas to criminalize homosexuality on the grounds of "protecting public health," put pressure on the White House to have donors sign a form that would make them criminally liable if their blood was found in the future to be contaminated with the AIDS factor.

When the White House approached the American Association of Blood Banks, this proposal was received with alarm, categorically rejected, and threatened to become a political embarrassment. Returning from a speaking engagement, Edward Brandt, who was unaware of the White House proposal, was paged in the Dallas airport by a White House staffer and frantically entreated to try to calm the blood bank officials.

Brandt, too, was appalled by the proposal. According to some observers, he agreed to intercede but only if he could tell the association that the proposal had originated with an unin-formed White House staffer and was not to be taken seriously.

The concerns of both the blood banking groups and fright-ened citizens continued to underscore the urgent need for reliable laboratory tests to screen for blood which contained the infectious agent that caused AIDS, and which could identify those people who had been exposed to that agent. Within two months, independent events were to add another dimension to the AIDS picture—scientific breakthroughs on the elusive virus, and the identification of yet another group of AIDS victims.

Scientific Success and Strife

On April 23, 1984, Secretary of Health and Human Services Margaret Heckler held a press conference in Washington, D.C., to announce a major breakthrough in attempts to control the AIDS epidemic and proclaim "the triumph of science over a dread disease." Often subsequently misquoted, Heckler's for-mal statement read:

Today I am proud to announce that the arrow of funds, medical personnel, research and experimentation which the Department of Health and Human Services and its allies around the world have aimed and fired at the disease AIDS has hit the target . . .

First, the probable cause of AIDS has been found—a variant of a known human cancer virus, called HTLV-III . . . Second, . . . a new process has been developed to mass produce this virus . . . Third, . . . we now have a blood test for AIDS which we hope can be widely available within about six months. We have applied for the patent on this process today . . . Finally, we also believe that the new process will enable us to develop a vaccine to prevent AIDS. We hope to have such a vaccine ready for testing in about two years.

The credit belongs to many people . . . In particular, credit should go to Dr. Robert Gallo, chief of the NCI laboratory of Tumor Cell Biology, who directed the research that produced this discovery; to Dr. Edward Brandt, the Assistant Secretary for Health who has led the

PHS-wide effort; to Dr. Vincent DeVita, Director of the NCI; and to Drs. James Mason and James Curran of the Centers for Disease Control.

And as is so often the case in scientific pursuit, other discoveries have occurred in different laboratories—even in different parts of the world . . . I especially want to cite the efforts of the Pasteur Institute in France, which has in part been working in collaboration with the National Cancer Institute. They have previously identified a virus which they have linked to AIDS patients, and within the next few weeks we will know with certainty whether that virus is the same one identified through the NCI's work. We believe it will prove to be the same.

Secretary Heckler's announcement coincided with the publication of results from Robert C. Gallo's laboratory at the National Cancer Institute. These studies identified the human T-cell lymphotropic virus, type III (HTLV-III) as the cause of AIDS. Gallo's reports were presented in four detailed and extensive papers, published back-to-back in *Science*.[27] These papers briefly alluded to the findings of a French group working with an isolate, called Lymphadenopathy Associated Virus (LAV), that had been described the year before in a *Science* article of May 1983.[28]

In retrospect, perhaps the gala press conference to announce the discovery of HTLV-III was not so unusual. In the mid-1950s Dr. Thomas Francis of the University of Michigan directed the first field trials of polio vaccine. Francis, with Jonas Salk at his side, announced the results on nationwide television.[29] Since then, scientific breakthroughs have become routine press conference material—for example, the cloning of an interferon gene[30] or a heart transplant operation. Yet Heckler's announcement differed because it carried the authority of the federal government.

Some of Secretary Heckler's predictions were later to have political consequences. The first, that a blood test based on the virus would become available within six months, proved only slightly optimistic, for HTLV-III blood-screening tests were ready for testing about nine months later. However, the legal, ethical, social and political questions concerning the use of the AIDS virus antibody test had only begun.

The second prediction was that a vaccine would be ready for testing in about two years, despite the lack of scientific precedence for such optimism. At the time of the press conference, no successful vaccine had ever been developed for any virus of the general type that included the AIDS-causing HTLV-III. The two-year target for vaccine production was apparently based on Gallo's opinion.[31]

Secretary Heckler also alluded to the work of Luc Montagnier and his group at the Pasteur Institute in France. Indeed, the press conference was closely followed by a series of television interviews at which Gallo and Montagnier appeared together, through satellite communication. Both men agreed that if the French LAV and American HTLV-III viruses were identical, this would simplify the development of diagnostic tests and vaccines. If they were different, then the number of viruses that could cause AIDS would have to be determined. A parallel in the history of polio was the discovery that three different types of virus caused the disease. Thus the polio vaccine had to be effective against all three. The answer to the question of whether LAV and HTLV-III were the same was of fundamental importance to Heckler's predictions. And if they turned out to be the same, perhaps the virus should be called by the French name. The debate over nomenclature was symptomatic of a growing rivalry between scientists working on the AIDS problem.

In a *New York Times* interview one day before Heckler's press conference,[32] James Mason, the CDC director-designate, described collaborative work on LAV by scientists at CDC and the French. His comments were taken to favor the French and to hint that CDC couldn't work well with the scientists at the NCI. In fact, Mason had only commented that data obtained at the CDC concerning antibodies to LAV were encouraging, and that these data supported the idea of retroviral etiology for AIDS. His statements were not directed at the growing controversy over who first discovered the AIDS agent. Indeed, knowledgeable CDC officials privately claimed that at the time he gave the interview, Dr. Mason had not yet been fully briefed on the NCI-Pasteur Institute controversy. Perhaps the eagerness with which Mason's remarks were received within the scientific community was because they appeared to document what so many had suspected—intra-agency rivalries.

Secretary Heckler's third prediction—that the extent of LAV/HTLV-III similarity would be known within a few weeks—was overly optimistic. Almost eight months passed before a detailed molecular comparison could be made of LAV and HTLV-III in early 1985. Meanwhile, reports that a third virus was independently isolated from AIDS patients came from the laboratory of Jay Levy at the University of California in San Francisco. These results, often overlooked, presaged what examination of a growing number of viruses recovered from AIDS patients would show, that virtually each AIDS virus isolate was unique.

Despite the intense interest and speculation on the part of the press and scientific community, neither Gallo nor Montagnier would comment on the extent of similarity between LAV and HTLV-III. Both the French and American groups had filed applications with the U.S. Patent and Trademark Office for the development of diagnostic tests using LAV and HTLV-III, respectively. The Montagnier group had applied for a U.S. patent in December 1983 (it was never awarded) for its work on a test to detect antibodies to the AIDS virus. The American group filed a patent application for an antibody detection test, as well as for a method for growing the virus in culture, five months later in April 1984. When the U.S. Patent and Trademark Office awarded a patent to the Americans in May 1985, the French group filed suit against the U.S. government in December 1985, alleging misappropriation of its technology. In June 1986, the Patent Office reversed itself and found that the French had priority in the discovery of the AIDS virus; in July the U.S. Claims Court ruled the additional claims of the French to royalties might be obviated by additional complications.[33] Lawyers for the Pasteur Institute declared an intent to appeal this decision, and in March 1987 the Federal Circuit Court revised the earlier Claims Court decision.[34] This long-standing dispute was finally resolved in an unprecedented way. On March 30, 1987, an agreement was signed between the U.S. Department of Health and Human Services and the Pasteur Institute to share rights and royalties to patent applications filed before May 25, 1985, with 80 percent of the royalties going to establish a foundation devoted to research on AIDS and other human retroviruses. This thoroughly unprecedented agreement was announced jointly by President Ronald Reagan and French Prime Minister Jacques Chirac, and marked the first time that the U.S. president publicly discussed AIDS. The document also contained a "chronology" (see Appendix A), which annotated the course of AIDS research that had been developed by Gallo and Montagnier and, again without precedent, was published in *Nature*.[35]

Following the public announcements, the energy that should have shifted to the challenge of translating the newly found etiologic agent into useful clinical tools was diverted to the courts and the political arena. The question of intellectual property rights also became a political weapon for those chagrined with the government's response to AIDS. The *New York Native*, a major homosexually oriented newspaper, devoted an issue to what it named "AIDSgate"[36]; the paper called for a congressional investigation of Gallo's claim to the discovery and naming of the AIDS virus, suspecting that the purpose of the announcement was to acknowledge the American group's preeminence in AIDS research, which would lead to increased support of its efforts. Although the *Native* may well have overstated its claim of being the champion of bringing the LAV/HTLV-III controversy into public view,[37] its coverage was certainly blunt and opinionated. Its accusations were directed not only at Gallo, the White House, and the PHS, but at the entire scientific community as well. The *Native* seemed to see Gallo's claim to discovering the cause of AIDS as a metaphor for federal management of the health crisis—that is, working on the basis of badly chosen priorities.

The controversy over who discovered the AIDS virus provides an illuminating glimpse of the rivalries and ambitions that beset the progress of biomedical research,[38] and it shows how public opinion can be shaped. Other scientific rivalries have been well publicized, among them the Pauling–Watson/Crick[39] race to discover the genetic importance of the structure of DNA, the long-standing Sabin–Salk[40] dispute over the contribution of each to the eradication of polio, and the ongoing rivalry of neurobiologists Schally and Guilleman, who shared a Nobel Prize for their work on neurohormones.[41] However, the story of the provenance and naming of the AIDS virus introduced a new element: the role of the federal establishment as an interested party. Margaret Heckler's optimistic announcement—an effort to communicate information during a novel health crisis—led to unanticipated complications, which, in turn, raised deeper and broader questions.

The entire public health approach to the AIDS crisis—working on developing a vaccine, planning a national information campaign, and allocating resources for research—for some time hinged on one question: were the viral strains isolated from AIDS victims identical? This basic scientific question was obscured by attention to allegations—like those of the *Native*—that Heckler's announcement of HTLV-III as the AIDS virus was made for political reasons. The controversy directed public attention away from the CDC's epidemiologic work and created the false impression that the research period had ended, when in fact it had just begun. Yet despite the colorful coverage by the *New York Native*, concerns about how well the system governing scientific research functions—a system that has continually resisted public oversight—are serious and deserve attention.

Regardless of the *political* settlement concerning who discovered the AIDS virus, and who will garner the Nobel prizes or public opprobrium, the May 1984 acceptance of HTLV-III/LAV as the cause of AIDS irreversibly changed the nature of managing the epidemic. Prior to that time AIDS research was groping: now it had direction. Scientists could go on to real targeting of specific tests and treatment and prevention strategies. Whereas coordination and augmented resources had always been desirable, they now became mandatory. And so the debate over research management strategies as well as questions of public policy was dramatically changed.

The Congressional Hearings

Edward Brandt's labeling of AIDS as the Public Health Service's "number one priority" in 1983 did more than catch public attention: it spurred congressmen Ted Weiss (D-New York) and Henry Waxman (D-California) to organize congressional hearings on the issue. The immediacy of the AIDS problem for Ted Weiss's New York City constituency, and the oversight responsibility of the subcommittee he chaired (Intergovernmental Relations and Human Resources Subcommittee of the Committee on Government Operations) argued for him to take an aggressive stand in investigating the efforts of HHS in the AIDS crisis. As for Waxman, his constituency in Los Angeles was as sensitive as any to AIDS, and he had long been a major spokesman on issues of health. Waxman chaired the Committee on Science and Technology of the House Energy and Commerce Committee.[42] Both subcommittees proceeded to hold hearings, and the Weiss subcommittee simultaneously asked the Government Accounting Office (GAO) to audit the books at both the CDC and NIH. The two subcommittees jointly requested a study by the Office of Technology Assessment (OTA).

The debate on Capitol Hill centered on whether the administration was committing appropriate resources to research the disease. "Too little and almost too late" is how Henry Waxman characterized research efforts at the August 1983 hearings on the federal response to AIDS. "Too little Aid for AIDS" screamed an August 1984 headline in *Technology Review*. In response to these kinds of criticism, Edward Brandt noted:

The basic issue is, should more money have been spent on AIDS? Would it have moved the research process any faster? . . . I continue to believe that during the first three years of this epidemic we had enough money to deal with the scientific aspects of this disease in a rational, thoughtful and orderly fashion.[43]

The early oversight hearings on AIDS were important because they provided a public forum for executive and congressional positions. In looking back on his participation as the public official then most directly charged with the AIDS effort, Brandt considered it his role "to put forth publicly our comprehensive plan for dealing with this epidemic and to respond to virtually all of the charges that had been made by the various groups. The press coverage from that hearing was quite favorable and the panic began to subside."[44] On the other hand, Brandt's comprehensive plan was described by Ted Weiss as "sort of hit or miss."[45]

Although the PHS and congressional critics disagreed on whether the federal strategy for managing the public health emergency was adequate, they knew the public watched the congressional inquiry closely, and its reaction would affect management of the government's programs. If the congressional hearing is political theater, the congressional actors are often playing to a home audience.

In April 1983 the Weiss subcommittee, through staffers Susan Steinmetz and Jim Mitchy, formally requested the services of the GAO to perform an audit of CDC and NIH regarding their AIDS activities. According to Martin Landry, an experienced GAO auditor who was eventually detailed to the subcommittee, the effectiveness of three CDC programs to be assessed were AIDS surveillance, AIDS laboratory studies, and AIDS epidemiology. On the surface, this was standard fare for the GAO. For example, Landry had performed audits of CDC's Agent Orange and Superfund efforts.

Landry—like most auditors—had no substantial knowledge of CDC programs. Yet this was not a problem, because the evaluative criteria were not meant to be technical. Rather, the audit would attempt to determine "self-consistency" of the agency's stated plans through an examination of the documents in the files. Landry would look to see if epidemiologic studies listed as high priority in planning documents had been performed, and if not, why not. Although Landry's approach reflected GAO policy and appeared logical, it was flawed in this case. For it is only with technical competency that one can adequately judge whether "self-consistency" occurs. It has been suggested that a more useful auditing procedure would have been a joint venture between the GAO and agency personnel, like one employed in the case of Reye's Syndrome. But the acrimony eventually generated during the AIDS audit precluded such cooperation.[46]

A preliminary fact-finding trip by Susan Steinmetz to Atlanta in May 1983 ended in an unprecedented manner: Director William Foege ordered her to leave CDC premises. The audit itself did not begin until three months later, after an often heated exchange of accusations and counterarguments between Weiss on the one hand and Foege and Heckler on the other. From Landry's perspective, the acrimony resulted from the attitude of the subcommittee in commissioning the audit: Weiss and his staffers suspected that the executive branch was concealing information and perhaps minimizing the epidemic, and the audit in Atlanta was therefore a hunt for a smoking gun.[47] Also contributing to the climate in Atlanta that initially precipitated these events were personality differences, as well as congressional distrust of the PHS's management of the AIDS problem.

The CDC's director, William Foege, displays a steely acumen where his work is concerned. A religious man, he served as a missionary medical officer a decade before becoming director of the CDC during the Carter administration.[48] Foege enjoys an exemplary reputation both as a public health officer and as an open and friendly individual. Susan Steinmetz is stylish and energetic with a no-nonsense, aggressive approach to her work. Those who know Foege agree that his asking her to leave was an uncharacteristic expression of frustration and irritation, a measure of last resort.

The crux of the friction was that the CDC and Weiss weighed the factors of patient confidentiality and congressional oversight differently. In his first letter to Foege following the Atlanta debacle, Weiss held that he had the right of access to all CDC personnel and files. The refusal of the CDC to open its files was seen as evidence of the administration's obfuscation. On the other hand, Secretary Heckler, supporting Foege's decision to protect CDC medical records, noted that HHS was restricted by law from allowing access to files containing patient-specific information.[49]

The principle of confidentiality surrounding medical records has a long tradition. Preservation of the confidentiality of the physician-patient relationship, and by extension, the researcher-subject relationship, is considered critical to providing the highest quality of medical care. Foege's vigilance in preserving the confidentiality reflected commonly held professional ethics in public health that emphasize respect for an individual's privacy.

One irony of the AIDS experience was that superb voluntary participation by the homosexual community in epidemiologic studies of hepatitis B virus vaccine had provided information that was crucial to the rapid understanding of how AIDS was spread. The personal and professional risk of being identified as homosexual, and therefore as an AIDS target, was of great concern to those asked to participate in these studies, and the CDC was committed to protect their privacy, in part because disclosure could well have derailed the agency's efforts. It was on this issue that Foege refused the subcommittee free access to the agency files, which did contain information that could identify the patients.[50]

Correspondence continued in this vein for another two months, with Weiss stressing his subcommittee's oversight authority and Foege maintaining the need for medical research and moral integrity.[51] The two sides finally agreed that the CDC would give GAO auditor Landry any file, but with all patient identifiers removed.

Foege returned to Atlanta following the August hearings and called a meeting at CDC to introduce Landry and the audit. According to Landry, at the meeting the CDC's executive officer was reported to have said that Landry should not be allowed to ask CDC personnel the question, "What else could have been done?"—something the subcommittee had said it needed. It looked as if the investigation was about to be derailed once again. Landry, reporting back to the subcommittee, found an enraged Weiss about to leave for a trip to Africa. In short order Weiss called Brandt, who called Foege, who worked out the last wrinkle.[52]

While Landry was performing the CDC audit, Steinmetz directed a simultaneous audit of NIH activities. The results of both investigations were summarized in a report that included a dissenting opinion signed by ten Republican members of the thirty-nine-member subcommittee,[53] who found the report to be without "substance and direction."

The report focused its criticism on administration funding problems and system-wide logistic delays. There was no evidence of an AIDS smoking gun. The Weiss report cited management problems in coordination, funding, and communicating within PHS, but offered no solutions. Nevertheless, the areas selected for criticism deserve attention, for no party disputed that such problems existed or that they awaited resolution.

2

Monitoring Public Health

THE INSTITUTIONS that constitute the health establishment perform medical research, monitor and survey public health, and deliver health services. Of these three functions the activities of those who oversee the public's health are the most political. For example, youngsters cannot register for school without proof of vaccination against childhood diseases. Although generally not seen as controversial in the 1980s, mandatory vaccination has had a stormy history illustrative of the tension between individual freedoms and the social restrictions that the public health enterprise devises to protect the common good. Other public health activities such as surveillance of disease, quarantine, inspection of restaurants, and so on, have high visibility and often engender dispute.[1]

The contemporary American public health establishment traces its origins to 1798 with the passage of the Act for the Relief of Sick and Disabled Seamen, which provided medical care to sailors and called for a hospital to be built for that purpose. This act was one of the earliest federal activities that was not related directly to the operation of government.[2] Its intent was less to care for the sick sailor than to protect against the entry of disease via sailors arriving in the United States. Fiscal support came not from general revenues but from a tax of 20 cents per months on seamen's wages, reflecting taxation only of those who were to benefit from the service. From these origins, hospitals and clinics evolved in port cities and became the first federal health-care delivery institutions.

Politics affected the choice of a director for the Boston Marine Hospital, established under the 1798 act. In 1804 President John Adams was about to appoint the director. A leading contender for the position was his schoolmate, Dr. Benjamin Waterhouse, an early and vocal advocate of smallpox vaccination. Because of the controversial nature of the issue, Adams decided not to appoint Waterhouse but instead chose a candidate opposed to widespread vaccination. In reviewing the history of the period, Dr. Jesse Steinfeld (surgeon general from 1969-1973) has attributed Adams's decision to the president's personal views. As head of the American Academy of Arts and Sciences, Adams listened to the debate about endorsing smallpox vaccination, but was not convinced by Waterhouse's arguments.

Three years later, in 1807, Thomas Jefferson, himself a scientist, succeeded Adams as president and subsequently appointed Waterhouse to the hospital's directorship. Waterhouse, who proceeded to champion vaccination, was later accused of setting up a monopoly on the distribution of the smallpox vaccine. President James Madison, Jefferson's successor, ultimately fired Waterhouse. Steinfeld draws three lessons from this anecdote:

First, the two Presidents [Adams and Jefferson] concerned with its [the hospital] creation were knowledgeable, and personally involved in the health affairs of the new nation. They could act and make decisions on the basis of personal knowledge rather than on staff advice filtered through layers of political appointees. Second, the early United States politics was not a "dirty business" for physicians, scientists, and medical professors but rather a matter of deep concern and personal involvement for all. And third, if the second principle was to be effective, physicians had to eschew personal gain through politics lest their credibility be lost and their motives questioned.[3]

Conflicts generated by adherence to Steinfeld's principles remain characteristic of the public health enterprise.

Public Responsibility for Health

In the initial period of U.S. history, up to the Civil War, the health needs of Americans were met almost exclusively by the private sector. Gradually, though, public health—in large part defined as sanitation—began to be seen as an appropriate public responsibility. And the distribution of services among health institutions developed as a patchwork of federal, state, and local programs. An important source of current tension in the American health establishment is this division of responsibility among federal, state, and local public health officials, coupled with the uneven pace of institutional change.

From the time of the act establishing the marine hospitals through the nineteenth and early twentieth centuries, infectious diseases constituted the majority of public health problems. Yet the control of communicable diseases was left to the authority of individual states. Despite increasing knowledge of the spread of infectious diseases and a growing need for an organized and centralized public health effort, it was not until seventy-two years later that Congress[4] formally organized the Marine Hospital Service as a national agency with a central headquarters and with a supervisory surgeon in charge of its hospitals.[5]

The 1870 Act (16 Stat. L. 169) was Congress's solution to a number of problems caused by marine hospitals that were poorly located and underfunded. Supplemental funds had to be appropriated continuously to provide service. Most problematic was the absence of a central supervisory authority. Until the 1870 Act was passed, the responsibility for running the service belonged to the president, who delegated it to the secretary of the treasury, who had no mechanism to centralize or coordinate its activities. Under the 1870 Act, the surgeon general of the Marine Hospital Service was given congressional authority to impose quarantines within the United States. This marked the first time that the federal government assumed public health responsibility in an area where the states had previously held jurisdiction.[6]

Subsequent progress in that direction was so uneven and slow that on the occasion of America's bicentennial Lister Hill could still point to certain persisting patterns:

It was only in our own twentieth century . . . that the federal government began to take a more active interest in medicine and the public health . . . first, through an attack upon the immediate threat of epidemic diseases . . . second, through measures of quarantine and sanitation reform . . . and third, through a hesitant and parsimonious use of the public treasure. I think that, upon reflection, we might all agree that these attitudes of the Congress eighty to one hundred years ago would be recognized among members of the House and Senate right up to today [1976]—and that these attitudes have been and still are present within the general body politic of America.[7]

The move to centralize health authority within the federal bailiwick was shaped by both the pragmatic need for centralized and coordinated action during epidemics of disease and by political desires to retain health authority at the local level. These conflicting drives, which continue to define the ambiguous division of public health responsibilities, were apparent in the management of cholera and yellow fever in 1878. Shortly after the consolidation of the marine hospitals,

after new cholera and yellow fever outbreaks, Congress gave the Marine Hospital Service authority to quarantine vessels that might be carrying contagious disease, but it also gave local authorities power to override any quarantine decision. When yellow fever struck New Orleans later that year, other public health reformers used the opportunity to induce Congress in March 1879 to establish a National Board of Health. This move, however, antagonized the Surgeon General, who four years later succeeded in persuading Congress to terminate the board. Thereafter, public health remained almost entirely a state and local responsibility.[8]

The absence of federal involvement did not prevent information about medicine and public health from expanding tremendously. Much of the knowledge gained was in the area of sanitation reforms; their implementation eliminated many problems that had previously been major public health concerns. For example, in 1900 tuberculosis, diarrhea, enteritis, and ulceration of the intestines were among the leading causes of death; in 1978 none of these was at the top.[9]

The Centers for Disease Control

Although authority for public health actions, such as closing restaurants and bath houses and stipulating vaccination in schools, still lies with state and local officials, the federal government today plays a critical role in monitoring public health. No single authority oversees all health research institutions, however. The majority of federal health activities fall within the purview of the Department of Health and Human Services (HHS); see Figure 1. Within this department the Public Health Service (PHS) and the Health Care Financing Administration (HCFA) are most involved in the federal response to a novel health emergency, at the same time remaining organizationally independent of each other. The PHS is composed of a number of agencies, including the Food and Drug Administration (FDA), National Institutes of Health (NIH), Centers for Disease Control (CDC), and the Alcohol, Drug Abuse and Mental Health Administration (ADAMHA). For practical purposes, these agencies plus the Veterans Administration (VA) and biomedical research laboratories within the Department of Defense make up the current federal health research establishment. The federal agency that provides epidemiologic and pragmatic guidance for local action is the CDC.

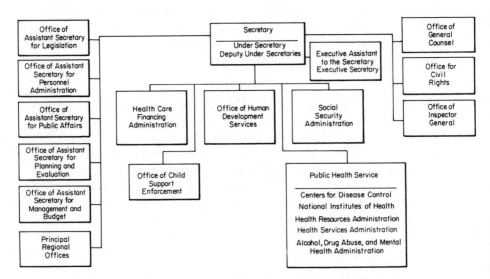

Figure 1. Department of Health and Human Services

The organization that grew into the CDC emerged during World War II as a malaria control program. Established and based in Atlanta, Georgia, where malaria was endemic, this agency evolved into the Communicable Disease Center in 1946 with an expanded mandate to track the incidence and trends of communicable diseases. The CDC's mission was enlarged even further to include surveillance and monitoring efforts for certain noninfectious diseases (workplace and environmental diseases, such as asbestosis and black-lung disease). In recognition of the growth of the agency's responsibilities, the CDC changed its name in 1970 (but kept its initials) to the Center for Disease Control. Following yet another reorganization, CDC became the Centers for Disease Control in 1980. The CDC currently consists of five centers and the National Institute for Occupational Safety and Health (NIOSH). Responsibilities include the training of epidemiologic and health workers, disease surveillance, licensing of clinical laboratories and laboratory tests involved in interstate commerce, and the conduct of research related to its mandate. The growth of CDC's activities is reflected in its budget: in FY85 Congress appropriated $410 million for CDC programs to be carried out by a total of 4,305 employees (Figure 2).

Epidemiology is central to the surveillance and monitoring mission of the CDC, and it is vital to establishing the research agenda during a novel health emergency. Traditionally, the distinction between basic and applied biomedical research has been used to differentiate research performed at the National Institutes of Health (NIH) from that done at the CDC. This too-often artificial distinction has long been a source of tension between the two agencies. NIH sees itself as the repository for basic biomedical research and views CDC as being engaged in applied work. Yet in the initial period of the AIDS emergency the work performed at the NIH to find the AIDS virus was the same as that done at CDC. NIH work was done under the rubric of basic research; at the CDC it was called epidemiology.

The initial period of research on AIDS illustrates a generic problem caused by overlapping activities of separate agencies.

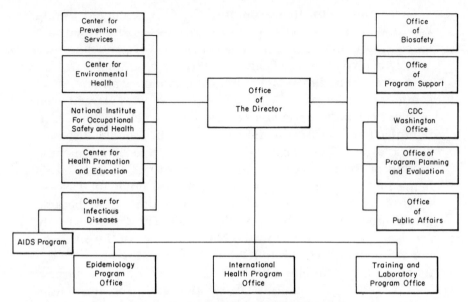

Figure 2. Centers for Disease Control

In December 1986 the CDC employed 4,138 people (including field staff), 192 of whom were working full time on AIDS. AIDS-related activities took place in the Center for Prevention Services, the Center for Health Promotion and Education, the Training and Laboratory Program, and the Center for Infectious Diseases (CID). The CID conducted AIDS research in the Hospital Infections Program, the Division of Host Factors, the Division of Parasitic Diseases, the Division of Viral Diseases, and the AIDS Program. The AIDS Program contains five branches: the Technical Information Activity, the Epidemiology Branch, the Statistics and Data Management Branch, the Surveillance Branch, and the Laboratory Branch.

Sources: Centers for Disease Control, and "Independent Assessment of Management and Productivity of the AIDS Program Laboratory of the CDC," a report by the Institute of Medicine, Division of Health Sciences Policy, December 1986.

The origin of the CDC-NIH interagency tension, says Dr. Alexander D. Langmuir, may be attributed to the establishment at CDC of epidemiologic surveillance programs that included research to determine the cause of outbreaks of disease.

The issue with NIH was long lived and sometimes bitter. NIH officials rightly claimed that over the previous half-century the National Hygienic Laboratory had a brilliant record of investigating epidemics and providing solutions . . . We at CDC countered with our new congressional charter that charged the agency with serving the states in the control of communicable disease, which certainly included the provision of epidemic aid on request. When the NIH officials were asked if they would accept responsibility for answering all such requests, they replied, "Certainly not. Only the interesting ones."[10]

Another administrator recalled that during the first year of the AIDS experience CDC and NIH worked harmoniously and "hand in glove" as equals. But in the second year, when the disease appeared to be perhaps the most important medical challenge of the century, the NIH argued that it should direct the research effort. The traditional interagency conflict between NIH and CDC surfaced anew. Similar research functions occurring in two different PHS agencies need not necessarily result in conflict: in fact, replication and independent confirmation of results is a hallmark of science. But during a crisis, when time is essential and materials limited, such efforts need to be coordinated.

Even the CDC's geographic distance from Washington has been discussed as a factor in interagency coordination. Although it has been suggested that physical separation can help insulate the agency from some of the political maneuvering that can consume other federal programs with headquarters in Washington,[11] during an emergency communication problems are better avoided.

The reorganization of CDC in 1980 illustrates the way organizational change can affect the flexibility of a health agency's response to an unanticipated emergency. At any particular time, the details of CDC's daily efforts reflect current disease outbreaks. Therefore reallocation of resources within CDC is the usual way to tailor the agency's resources to changing disease patterns. Before 1980, CDC's capabilities for laboratory and epidemiologic studies were organized along technical lines into discrete, agency-wide divisions. To improve its ability to redirect work, CDC reorganized so that each of the five centers would have laboratory and epidemiologic capabilities. The reorganization ended the bureaucratic separation of functions needed by each of the centers and was thought to facilitate reallocation efforts among categories of disease, rather than among types of technical services.

During the 1970s, under the leadership of William Foege, the CDC mission was likewise enlarged, to include wellness and health promotion. As these concepts became incorporated into CDC activities, they required that public education be given greater emphasis. In Foege's words:

Health-care services and health promotion are held to different standards, play by different rules . . . I view this dichotomy between health-care services and prevention techniques in the United States as absurd. The basic social value is that health is a priority, but attend to it only after you have lost it.[12]

At the time they were needed, the mechanisms for truly effective public information and education were not in place. The way information about AIDS was disseminated at large bears out Foege's comment. Little research was done on how best to provide sex education and to encourage change in sexual behavior. The attempt to provide information to the public about AIDS and its prevention was late to develop and was often left to those outside government. Despite Foege's goal, the government did not give any agency a clear assignment of the responsibility for public health education, accompanied by sufficient resources to implement educational programs, when AIDS surfaced in the early 1980s. The epidemic was to enter its sixth year before AIDS education became a sufficiently potent political issue to attract a significant congressional appropriation.

Federal, State, and Local Responsibilities

The historic assignment of health service responsibility is reflected in the complicated relations among different levels of government. The Constitution makes no explicit assignment of a health care function to the Congress. On the contrary, protection of the public health was implicitly reserved to the individual states as part of their police powers.[13]

In general, the functions of state governments are the establishment of state-wide health and the supervision of local public health. Seldom do state agencies provide services directly; local (city and county) public health departments provide most of the direct services. The federal government, which has increasingly financed health services since the 1930s, sets national policy through the establishment of budget priorities.

The Social Security Act of 1935 is generally acknowledged to have fostered current health service relations by initiating direct grants-in-aid for health to the states. That legislation provided an economic lever for the federal government to dominate state and local health services, and therefore the institutions available for response to health emergencies.

The functions appropriate for local health departments have been a continuing subject for discussion within the public health community. Reports issued by professional organizations such as the American Public Health Association (APHA) indicate the changing attitudes. In 1945 an APHA committee report enunciated standards for minimally adequate public health services to be provided by local health departments.[14] Six functions were listed: (1) vital statistics;[15] (2) communicable disease control; (3) sanitation,—which meant supervision of milk, water, and eating places; (4) laboratory services (Wassermann tests for syphilis, for example); (5) maternal and child hygiene, including school health program supervision; and (6) health education.

These "basic six" are all preventive activities, designed to control acute infectious diseases. However, by the 1970s perceptions had changed regarding what the "real" public health problems were, and what services local public health departments should provide. The change was due to widespread, successful implementation of sanitary engineering recommendations, improvements in the medical practice in controlling infectious disease, and increased public awareness of noninfectious causes of disease, thanks to efforts of the growing biomedical research community. The change in attitudes about public health services paralleled the shift of focus, almost twenty years earlier, in the research community, from infectious diseases of the young to chronic diseases of the aging. Thus public health authorities were now seen to be responsible for the care and control of chronic and degenerative diseases.

Additionally, as part of the environmental movement of the 1960s, public attention focused on consumer protection and environmental control (air pollution and toxic waste, for example). These activities also began to be viewed as appropriate for consideration by local public health departments. The growing list of what were appropriate local health issues differed from locality to locality. Public health departments in large cities were pressed to take on primary health-care delivery, while suburban departments focused on environmental issues. Yet neither environmental control nor primary health care fit among the six functions set as standard for a local public health department in the 1940s. Although the mandates were growing, federal funds were still allocated only for the traditional services. Consequently, having less money to spend for more services, the local departments fell short in public standing and in their performance of both conventional and new roles.[16]

The new issues engaging local public health officials were often beyond their capabilities and resources, leading in the 1960s to the reassignment of some public health responsibilities away from the local authorities. Such reassignment inevitably decreased the resources available to local departments. That local public health concerns are in large part dictated by local circumstances has direct relevance for managing a health emergency. The needs of different localities vary with the nature of the population at risk.

Just as the American Public Health Association articulated its goals for local public health departments, it has also done so for state health agencies, listing four functions[17]: (1) health surveillance, planning, and program development; (2) promotion of local health coverage; (3) setting and enforcement of standards; and (4) providing health services (generally a supervisory role;

where there is no functioning local health department, the state may provide direct service).

These diverse state and local health responsibilities are served by a wide array of institutions. And each of the fifty states and seven territories, which provide guidance to localities for health care services, has a distinctive system. If a trend develops to bypass state agencies and develop direct ties between the federal agencies which fund health and the local dispenser, the pattern can become even more complicated. This pluralism contributes to the confusion involved in dealing with a health emergency.

A good illustration of the fragmentation of the health system is the process of reporting diseases. Initially, the possibility that a public health problem may be developing arises from anecdotal reports transmitted via an informal public health network to the federal CDC. When enough information is gathered to indicate a problem—and exactly when that occurs is a matter of debate—a disease may be made "reportable": that is, now when a physician learns of a person with the disease in question, he is required to report it to public health officials.

The formal decision that a disease be nationally reportable is made by the Conference of State and Territorial Epidemiologists. The CDC, the Public Health Service, or a state official may approach the conference to request that this be done. And although the conference has no statutory power, a disease will not become nationally reportable without its recommendation. On the other hand, under current procedures, only the states, through their police powers, can make a disease reportable. As there are fifty states, there are fifty different reporting procedures. State health authorities can require that private physicians, labs, or hospitals report to an appropriate authority that a patient has a certain disease; to which authority the information is reported varies. The state may request that the person reporting the disease file a copy of the state report—or file an independent report—with the CDC. Alternatively, state health officials may themselves relay the information to Atlanta (the information collected is not standardized). Diagnosis, clinical test results, the names and characteristics of an individual—some or all of this information may be requested by public health officials. It is the state that decides what will be collected.

The process by which each state makes a disease reportable also varies. The decision may be made by executive order, or legislation may be required. Thus some states can quickly decide to collect statistics on a disease, whereas in other states it can take months and even years. Furthermore, the mandate and will to ensure that reporting is consistent are highly variable.

It is up to the CDC to decide what information it wants from the individual states. Yet CDC has no authority to require reporting, nor can it impose penalties if its requests are not met. State compliance with a request by the Conference of State and Territorial Epidemiologists and with federal surveillance efforts is based on tradition and on a common goal—the furtherance of public health. Thus the process by which a disease becomes reportable, thereby allowing the collection of data needed to develop a national strategy, requires voluntary cooperation of myriad institutions, each using unique procedures.

The nature of public health monitoring and surveillance requires that individuals be asked for information that is normally confidential. This is one of several greatly contentious policy issues that have come up in connection with AIDS and are at the core of the public health enterprise: questions of privacy and of individual versus social rights. For example, the debate concerning the confidentiality of patient records, raised first in the discussion of making AIDS a reportable disease, has surfaced in virtually every stage of the AIDS experience.

Adding to the difficulty of elaborating a national policy is the question of implementing such a policy, given the divided responsibility among federal, state, and local officials. CDC has only an advisory role. The authority to act in public health matters is reserved to the states. Thus the difficulty in implementing nationwide policy during the AIDS epidemic—for example in the schools, or the proper use of blood screening tests—derives from the historic division of public health responsibilities.

Likewise, the overlapping of epidemiologic work with fundamental research in the early period of the epidemic created ambiguity and conflict among the public health and research communities about responsibility and resource allocations. The approaches and missions of these two parts of the health research establishment, traditionally separate, merged during the initial years of the AIDS emergency.

3

Biomedical Research Institutions

THE Public Health Service (PHS) was chartered in 1912 explicitly to engage in "investigations of the diseases of man and of the pollution of navigable streams."[1] Its charter, with direct recognition of the association between research and public health, is derived from several sources: the PHS's origin in the 1798 Marine Act and the emphasis after that date on sanitation as the primary control of disease; the creation of health services in large urban hospitals in the mid-1800s; and the introduction at the turn of the nineteenth century of the scientific method into American medicine, which made schools of medicine that emphasized research programs the focus of public health. The major federal biomedical research and public health institutions of the 1980s are organizationally linked in the PHS.

The National Institutes of Health (NIH), the Food and Drug Administration (FDA), and the Centers for Disease Control (CDC) have common historic origins in the Marine Hospital Service, which in 1887 established the Hygienic Laboratory to investigate bacterial diseases. The Hygienic Laboratory received an expanded mandate a few years later to test and license the manufacture of biological products such as serums, viruses, and antitoxins.[2] The laboratory's function was to perform the research, but it had no regulatory powers. The responsibility for regulation had been granted to the Department of Agriculture.

Separation of Research, Regulation, and Medical Care

The regulatory authority of the Department of Agriculture had been established with enactment of the 1906 Food and Drugs Act, a statute that was in no small measure a response to public concern about hazards associated with patent medicine and food. Upton Sinclair's novel/exposé, *The Jungle*, served as a catalyst for the Food and Drugs Act of 1906. As the Department of Agriculture began to carry out the provisions of the act, and as the costs of regulation mounted, its budget and personnel needs outgrew its resources. The secretary of agriculture argued for even greater separation of research and regulatory functions, in order to protect resources for both activities. In 1927 the Congress created the Food, Drug, and Insecticide Administration (eventually to be called FDA in 1937) to enforce the regulatory aspects of the 1906 law.

Muckraking journalists and consumer advocates continued to question the adequacy of federal regulations to assure safety of food and drugs. In response, New Deal legislation in this area was introduced in Congress in 1933. The comprehensive Federal Food, Drug, and Cosmetic Act became law in 1938, and it is to this day the basic governing statute for these products. The licensing, research, and regulation of foods, drugs, biologicals, cosmetics, and medical devices remain functions of the FDA.

Under the 1938 Act, the Food, Drug, and Insecticide Administration was transferred to yet another part of the federal bureaucracy, the Federal Security Agency, the progenitor of the Department of Health and Human Services.[3] Although the 1938 legislation centralized numerous federal research, regulatory, and public health activities in a single agency, the oversight of toxins, serum, and vaccines remained with NIH as a vestige of the Hygienic Laboratory's nineteenth-century charter. Only in 1972 did Congress transfer regulatory control over these biological products to FDA.[4]

The administrative shift that resulted in a centralized federal health establishment with the 1938 Act paralleled some important changes in the focus of the medical establishment. First was the emergence, following the introduction of the scientific method, of medical schools as a forum for discussing scientific matters involving public health.

The essential elements of the scientific method are a hypothesis, experimentation to test that hypothesis, and independent verification of the results. Once introduced, this method stimulated communication among scientists and resulted in expanded research activity. As a result, twentieth-century medicine became increasingly more aggressive in designing research projects to identify, prevent, and treat disease. These changes were profound. As Vernon Lippard, the former dean of the Yale School of Medicine, has noted:

It would be difficult for one who has not lived through this period to appreciate the extent to which the introduction of research on a large scale changed the character of American medical schools. By 1920 the more progressive schools were becoming scientifically oriented, and small amounts of research support were being provided by foundations. Research activity was stimulated largely by personal initiative rather than by institutional pressures. Throughout the next twenty years a growing interest in research became evident, as did corresponding increased rewards in prestige for those engaged.[5]

The second momentous event that led to the separation of research and medical care was the discovery of penicillin in 1928. Alexander Fleming's discovery ushered in the era of antibiotic drugs, and by the 1940s acute bacterial infectious diseases such as bacterial pneumonia were no longer prominent as a cause of death. Attention now began to focus on chronic diseases such as cancer and arthritis. Unlike bacterial diseases, which had been brought under control through sanitation and antibiotics, chronic illnesses were not responsive to known treatment. Basic research was therefore increasingly emphasized as the way to attack such problems. Lippard points to the growing separation between fundamental scientific efforts and clinical service, which became critical to the evolution of contemporary public health institutions:

In the 1920s, the basic sciences were taught by individuals who, although often not physicians, had an interest in clinical medicine and made an effort to relate their instruction to clinical problems. As they were relieved of clinically related responsibilities, they turned their attention to more fundamental issues.[6]

The presence of researchers and clinicians in the same institution should have fostered linkages. As information about the life sciences expanded and research became more sophisticated, however, the two groups specialized and moved farther apart.

The era of antibiotics and the enthusiasm for medical research coincided with a fortuitous political change: the election of Franklin Roosevelt and the emergence of New Deal political ideology. The shift in politics led to the government's assumption of numerous social initiatives, including public health efforts and medical research. Thus the Social Security Act of 1935 allowed direct federal support of research at the local level by initiating grants-in-aid to the states. This great innovation promoted the growth of a federal research establishment, because the new grant-giving ability opened the way and provided the means for direct federal intervention in research in nonfederal facilities.

The trend toward increasing federal involvement in health activities through explicit linking of research with health service continued with the establishment in 1937 of the National Cancer Institute. NCI's mandate was to determine the cause, prevention, and treatment of cancer, to coordinate the research effort of the institute and other research groups, and to work with state health agencies in the struggle against cancer.[7] The National Cancer Act gave the government the first permanent authority to grant federal funds for basic research to private institutions, thus encouraging the growth of university-based biomedical research. The federal commitment was subsequently bolstered with additional direct federal assistance to the states[8] in the form of additional grants-in-aid.[9]

While the statutes of the late 1930s and 1940s created direct channels between Washington and local research facilities, they simultaneously undermined other linkages. Communication between local scientists and their institutes and state authorities diminished as the federal establishment underwrote an increasing part of the research effort. Thus the research eventually moved away from monitoring, surveillance, and health-care delivery services, which remained state and local responsibilities.

Although the machinery for federal dominance of research was in place at that time, federal research support was only nascent. Thus when the National Foundation for Infantile Paralysis—a private, nonprofit foundation—was established in the late 1930s, its founders recognized that the research efforts would have to be supported by private funding.[10] Substantial federal assistance came only after the intensive, privately supported research had been organized and was successful. Close to thirty years later, however, the majority of biomedical research became federally supported. In 1956, when the first field trials of Salk polio vaccine were held, the federal budget for all research and development in health totaled $81 million (in current dollars). In contrast, $4.56 billion was spent in 1984.[11] The dramatic change in federal support and dominance of biomedical research cannot be overemphasized. For this reason, the conquest of polio as a model for research management strategies to meet public health emergencies such as AIDS is very limited.

In 1930 the Ransdell Act turned the Hygienic Laboratory into the National Institute of Health, giving it the expanded mandate to determine the cause, prevention, and cure of disease. NIH grew phenomenally. In 1980 it was composed of twelve institutes which supported biomedical research,[12] and included a clinical center and the Fogarty International Center. NIH supported the breadth of biomedical research with a total FY85 budget of $5.14 billion. Because of the nature of research, the paths followed within different NIH institutes often overlap, and the demarcation lines between medical research disciplines are understood to be fluid. Yet the association of a name of a field, like cancer or heart disease with an institute has great drawing power. Thus, between 1980 and 1985, proposals were introduced in Congress to establish no fewer than eleven additional new institutes at NIH and to transfer four existing health agencies to NIH.[13]

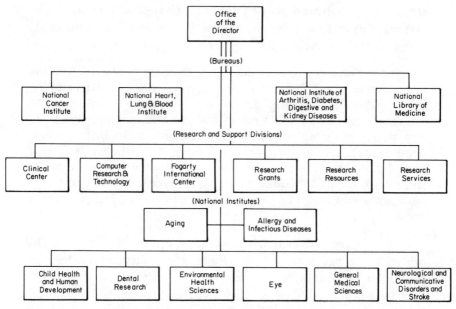

Figure 3. National Institutes of Health

In the period of broad government retrenchment of the eighties the Congress, the executive branch, and the NIH and special health lobbies pushed their own priorities for how the limited federal research dollar should be spent. For example, in the early 1980s extensive congressional debate centered on the creation of a new arthritis institute as well as an institute of nursing research. The director of NIH took the position that new institutes were not needed and would only deflect limited funds from research to administration. To bolster this position in a contentious debate, and in the hopes of eliminating "institute building" as a frequently used tactic, the NIH—in response to pressure from HHS—commissioned a study by the prestigious Institute of Medicine (IOM).[14]

The goal of the report was to develop criteria for future organizational changes in the NIH. In a summary and analysis of that study later written by the study's staff director and committee chairman, organizational change as a tactic for setting the national health research agenda was criticized. These authors concluded:

Organizational changes should not be the only means, or even the primary means for NIH to alter its research priorities . . . NIH and the Public Health Service need to develop new mechanisms to judge impartially the merits of proposed changes and more important, to find effective nonorganizational responses to emerging needs and opportunities. In the long run, we believe, the nation will be best served if NIH and the other agencies cooperate more with the public and the scientific community in setting research priorities and take a more active and visible role in finding ways to address health-research needs.[15]

This conclusion was reached with the understanding that "In our current political system, there are many advocates for particular aspects of health research but few for its entirety."[16] The traditional way in which advocacy positions for special health-research interests have been most effectively expressed has been through congressional mandate of budgetary and organizational change.

Budget and Organization of the NIH

Most basic biomedical research in the United States is funded, and therefore controlled, by the NIH. Its 1985 research budget accounted for 64 percent of the government's health research and development expenditures and 38 percent of the total national health budget. NIH's work was carried out by a staff of 14,413 located in its twelve institutes, its Division of Research Resources, the Fogarty Center, and the Clinical Center. Withal, only when we realize that over 80 percent of NIH's research funds are spent at nonfederal institutions can we appreciate the extent of the direct effect of NIH policy on the entire biomedical research community.

The NIH supports biomedical research through intramural and extramural programs. Intramural research is carried out principally in the NIH's own laboratories and in some outside laboratories that are under contract for specific requirements of the intramural scientists' experimentation (such as the production by Litton Bionetics in Frederick, Maryland, of HTLV-III, a virus isolated from patients with AIDS or AIDS-like symptoms). The extramural programs are carried out exclusively in non-government, usually university laboratories. Intramural and extramural programs differ in the way that research is selected, managed, and evaluated, in the extent and type of peer review, and in the role assigned to the two programs within the national biomedical research effort. The extramural activities are managed by program offices located in each of the NIH institutes.[17] The research is funded either through contracts initiated by the NIH with an outside investigator (targeted funds) or through grants requested by the investigator (nontargeted funds). Work supported by nontargeted funds is often mistakenly equated with basic research, and work supported under targeted programs is viewed as applied research. In fact, the distinction depends on how closely the NIH monitors the course of research (contract research is monitored more closely).

It is commonly believed in the biomedical research community that science advances best through individual initiative. Therefore, the investigator-initiated grant (ROI) system, which funds most nontargeted research, is the mechanism traditionally used to support basic research in universities. These ROI grants represent approximately 80 percent of the extramural budget, or approximately 60 percent of the total NIH research budget,[18] and have become the symbolic measure of the level of the nation's biomedical research effort.[19]

Individual ROI grants are reviewed and awarded through a two-tiered system designed to standardize criteria and quality across all NIH units; to allow individuality in setting priorities for research within individual institutes; and to draw on the collective scientific judgment of the research community. During the first-tier review, an investigator's proposal is reviewed by a "study section" composed of scientists from universities, industry, and the government.[20] If a proposal is approved for funding, it is given a ranking (100 highest rank, to 500 lowest rank) and is referred for second-tier review by the advisory council of the appropriate institute. The second-tier review places a research proposal within the context of an individual institute's programs.

The council is composed of outside consultants drawn from health care practitioners, scientists, and the lay public. It reviews each grant for relevance to the institute's research goals, and can modify the ranking (increase or decrease the score) to reflect the institute's priorities. The council can also adjust funding patterns to meet an institute's objectives by establishing different "pay-lines" for different areas of research. Each institute has a fixed budget for its extramural program. Therefore much of second tier review is establishing a "pay-line"—the level at which grants will be paid. For example, in FY83 and FY84, the National Institute of Allergy and Infectious Diseases (NIAID) funded grants with scores of 100-166 and 100-162, respectively. On the other hand, research in an area seen to be of particular relevance might have been paid at 250. In an analogy with the federal budgeting process, first-tier review is scientific authorization, and second-tier review is program appropriation.

Distribution of NIH research resources among the institutes is negotiated with the Congress. Each institute's budget, including the proportion of funds in intramural versus extramural programs, appears as a line item in the federal budget. Special health interest groups lobby on behalf of different institutes, and institute directors are frequently heard to describe their various "constituencies." In FY85 the largest institute budget was that of the National Cancer Institute ($1.18 billion); the smallest was at the Dental Research Institute ($100 million). The two largest institutes—NCI and Heart, Lung and Blood—accounted for 37 percent of the total NIH budget.

The intramural research programs represented approximately 12 percent of the NIH budget (FY83). This work—performed for the most part by civil servants—is overseen by the scientific director of each institute, acting in only loose coordination with other parts of NIH. Within each institute, the intramural agenda is established in consultation (but not necessarily agreement) of that institute's scientific advisers. Unlike the extramural program with its highly prescriptive peer review system, review within the intramural programs is more idiosyncratic, unstandardized, and varies among institutes.[21]

A health emergency is disruptive to the way extramural and intramural agendas are set. Whereas normally 80 percent of research funds go to extramural programs, in the early period of the AIDS crisis the bulk of federal AIDS research resources were expended in intramural programs. This was in large part because intramural research efforts could be redirected more quickly and easily. But as the AIDS epidemic and associated research budget mushroomed, more scientists turned to AIDS research and received extramural grants and contracts. So, for example, in 1985 the NIAID established a division of AIDS activities in its extramural program. The extramural programs AIDS budget for FY85 was $47.3 million, as compared with $13.8 million for the intramural AIDS effort. The amount allocated to NIAID's extramural AIDS programs looks even more dramatic when we realize that administrative and personnel costs for NIH employees who directed the extramural effort are included in the $13.8 million.

Who Sets the Research Agenda?

At NIH this fundamental policy issue can be seen as a series of decisions: determining the amount of research resources; distributing resources first between institutes (disease categories), and then within each institute by program priorities; within programs, distributing funds among intramural and extramural facilities; and eventually deciding which projects to support. Each of these questions became a point of controversy during the first years of the AIDS epidemic.

The research manager's goal is to achieve practical results, but the path selected may not yield those results. Research management is very much a gamble, and the successful manager is one who knows where to place the bet. The basic research scientist, on the other hand, most often believes that answers to specific medical problems can be found only in the study of fundamental biochemical mechanisms, addressed in the lab in systems that may seem unrelated to the disease in question. He believes, in short, that pragmatic results come from basic research. When a specific answer is needed to meet a health emergency, friction is likely to develop between the managers and the basic research scientists about how to perform the research. For example, when the National Foundation for Infantile Paralysis drew up a program that identified specific problems in polio research and targeted groups of scientists most capable of researching those problems, it met with strong opposition from scientists who considered such a focused approach to the causes and prevention of polio to be inappropriate.[22]

The question of whether disease-specific research can be targeted was also central to the debate around AIDS; indeed, it is a matter for discussion whether the missions of federal research institutions are compatible with targeted emergency efforts. These questions can be illustrated by an anecdote about targeting AIDS research at the National Cancer Institute. An early phenomenon that drew attention to AIDS was the epidemic occurrence of Kaposi's sarcoma. Before it was discovered that this cancer was a secondary complication of immune deficiency, there was concern that an epidemic of cancer might take place. The NCI, the federal institution charged by the Congress with cancer prevention and cure, developed a research strategy. The institute chose to focus on retroviruses, almost to the exclusion of other lines of research, for several reasons. First, some scientists felt the evidence for a retroviral cause of AIDS was strong. Second, a commitment to retrovirus research was well established at the NCI. After the causative role of a retrovirus was proved, an NCI official was queried about the wisdom of an "all the eggs in one basket" strategy as an emergency research policy. That official noted that if the gamble had failed, the effort would have been worthwhile anyway because basic retroviral research was a priority of the NCI. This comment points out how the priorities of the immediate crisis effort are often shaped by, or may be in conflict with, previously established program objectives.

Two aspects of the AIDS epidemic have made another public health agency, the Alcohol, Drug Abuse, and Mental Health Administration (ADAMHA), a player in behavioral research on AIDS. First, one group early identified to be at risk for AIDS was the IV drug abusers. Second, AIDS was and still is an incurable disease whose spread is best controlled by educating the public to avoid high-risk behavior. Research relevant to such educational efforts is concentrated within ADAMHA, which deals with diseases whose causes and treatment are characterized by behavioral change.

ADAMHA's antecedents can be traced to 1930, when the Division of Mental Hygiene was created within PHS for the treatment of narcotic addicts, and to 1946, when the National Mental Health Act established the National Advisory Council on Mental Health and a broad program of grants for research, training, and community mental health centers. The Division of Mental Hygiene was replaced by the National Institute of Mental Health (NIMH) in 1949.

The Community Health Services and Facilities Act and the Mental Health Centers Construction Act[23] resulted in major expansion of NIMH's activities. These services were further extended by the Narcotic Addict Rehabilitation act of 1966[24] and the Alcohol Abuse and Alcohol Prevention, Treatment, and Rehabilitation Act of 1970,[25] which also provided for the establishment of a National Institute on Alcohol Abuse and Alcoholism (NIAAA) within NIMH. The National Institute on Drug Abuse (NIDA) was formed within NIMH in 1972 with passage of the Drug Abuse Office and Treatment Act.[26] These three institutes—NIMH, NIDA, and NIAAA—were merged into ADAMHA by administrative order in May 1974, and the agency's status was subsequently clarified by statute.[27]

The organizational separation of ADAMHA from NIH illustrates the well-debated tendency of separating the social scientist's approach to understanding human behavior from basic biomedical research. The biomedical and social sciences have long been divorced from the perspective of federal support for research. For example, much social science research is supported by the National Science Foundation, an independent federal agency. When AIDS was defined as a PHS research problem, only part of the relevant federal research effort was found among its programs. It proved difficult to locate other federal resources and coordinate them with PHS programs.

In reviewing the prospects for funding domestic research programs in the 1980s, conventional wisdom holds that one way to support research is to hide a program in the defense budget. The biomedical research effort at the Department of Defense (DOD) is thought to be significant. Similarly, an independent federal agency with ties to DOD—the Veterans Administration—also figures in funding of federal biomedical research.

Although research represents only a small fraction of its budget ($192.4 million for FY85), the VA has a vast network of clinical research programs. In addition, many VA hospitals are affiliated with university medical centers. University researchers may be housed in VA facilities, while they do research supported by a NIH grant. Consequently, it is difficult to determine exactly what federal agency is supporting which research effort. Moreover, the VA is not administratively linked to the PHS, so there is no clear line of command if joint efforts are needed during an emergency. Although the FY87 budget called for a coordinated federal AIDS effort, the failure to link AIDS expenditures in HHS with those in the VA and the DOD precluded a truly effective coordination.

Another participant in medical services and research is a roster of nonprofit private foundations. These foundations in part provide support for research programs, but their major role is to serve as advocates for certain research efforts. The strong presence of these and other special-interest health lobbyists since World War II has given rise to the term "disease of the month" to indicate the pressure brought to bear on the Congress by advocates for specific diseases. Curiously, none of the established private funding organizations prominent in biomedical research championed the fight against AIDS early in the epidemic.[28] Rather, new foundations were established for this purpose, with only one—the American Foundation for AIDS Research (AMFAR)—achieving significant capital resources in the mid 1980s. In the AIDS crisis the most visible special-interest lobbies have been those of the gay rights organizations, the hemophilia society, and the blood banking industry (such as the American Red Cross and American Association of Blood Banks), and, eventually, AMFAR. In November 1984 a full-time countrywide lobbying effort for the Federation of AIDS-Related Organizations—the AIDS Action Council—came into being, exemplifying the growing political sophistication of AIDS activists.

In addition to lobbying, the special-interest groups and foundations play an important role in providing direct seed funding of research. Although most federal funds for medical research are distributed through the extramural programs of the National Institutes of Health, the time elapsed from preparation of the grant proposal to the actual receipt of funds can be as much as two years. In contrast, the flexibility of the smaller, less rigidly structured private foundations allows them to respond much more rapidly to a request for funds.

4

Delivering Health Care

Whereas the CDC dominates public health and the NIH dominates biomedical research, no single, federal institution has overall responsibility for patient care (save the VA, which serves only a fraction of the population). The pluralism that characterizes the health delivery system is staggering. As Paul Torrens observed:

There isn't any single "American health care system." There are many separate subsystems serving different populations in different ways. Sometimes they overlap; sometimes they are entirely separate from one another. Sometimes they are supported with public funds, and at other times they depend solely on private funds. Sometimes several different subsystems use the same facilities and personnel that are entirely separate and distinct.[1]

Traditionally, the term "medical care" has been used for care of individuals by or under the direction of a physician.[2] In recent years the term has expanded to refer to the general field of health care, including nursing, dentistry, physical therapy, and so on. The substitution of "health" for "medical" (or "patient") reflects the disagreement among health professionals as to who dominates the health care field.

During a health emergency services may be provided by (among others) community health nurses, health educators, nutritionists, optometrists, podiatrists, and pharmacists in such locations as hospitals and community centers.[3] Thus a health emergency involves a broad array of institutions, only a few of which are directly accountable to the federal government. The lack of demarcation of responsibility for health services profoundly affects the management of a new disease. Clinical research, together with epidemiologic surveys, tends to focus the efforts of the scientist at the bench. Yet questions of payment and assignment of responsibility for such research—clinical trials of new drugs and devices, use of existing therapeutics in a new setting—are uncharted areas without clear policy guidelines. Although virtually all care is experimental and can be accurately viewed as clinical research, the process by which the primary care physician participates in the emergency research effort is similarly vague.

Paying for Health Care

The pluralism that characterizes health care delivery extends not only to the institutional affiliation of a primary care provider, and to the kinds of practitioner, but also to the methods of payment. Although an increasingly large proportion of health care funding is provided by federal and state funds, a great deal is not. In 1983, for example, 41.9 percent of the total $355.4 billion in health care costs was accounted for by public funds. In contrast, in 1955, just before polio vaccine trials, 25.7 percent of that year's $17.7 billion bill (in 1983 dollars) came from public sources.[4] During an emergency, the omnipresent problem of who is responsible for paying for health care is further complicated by uncertainties of what constitutes "standard" care, for federal insurance pays only for established treatments.

For AIDS, the problem and the cost augmented as the epidemic spread. In early 1986, estimates of the average direct lifetime cost for caring for an AIDS patient at different places in the country ranged from $21,000 to $140,000.[5] At San Francisco General Hospital, the cost of treatment for a patient from the time of diagnosis to death varied from $50,000 to $100,000.[6] As the number of AIDS patients grew into the tens of thousands, the CDC estimated that the medical costs alone to the country of the first 10,000 would be $1.4 billion.

The Health Care Finance Administration (HFCA) has an increasing responsibility for AIDs programs. HCFA is an HHS agency independent of the PHS. Created in 1977 to bring Medicare, Medicaid, and related quality control programs under a single administrative unit, HCFA is responsible for funding long-term care. As the primary source of government funds for direct delivery of health care to the individual (such as money for hospitalization bills and disability insurance), HCFA is a critical part of the government's response to a novel health crisis.

Even after AIDS has been classified as a disabling disease—thereby paving the way for a patient to become eligible for Medicare—HCFA's rules were problematic. There was a statutory two-year period (in the early 1980s, that was the life expectancy for AIDS patients) between being classified as having a disabling disease and becoming eligible for receiving Medicare assistance. Even after this bureaucratic problem was resolved, HCFA rules remained an obstacle for reimbursing "experimental" treatments. Throughout 1986, there was no standard therapy for AIDS; all treatment was experimental.[7] For example, interferon began to be tested in AIDS patients in 1983 at the Sloan-Kettering Institute in New York and at San Francisco General Hospital. It was not proved effective, but even if it had been, HCFA would not pay for the treatment because interferon was an experimental drug.

HCFA was established as an independent agency during the Carter Administration, when Joseph Califano was Secretary of the Department of Health, Education and Welfare. HCFA's organization was deliberately designed to separate Medicare and Medicaid from the Social Security Administration as well as from the Public Health Service. In one interpretation, this move sprang from the desire to distance the economic power base in HHS (HCFA represents over 20 percent of the HHS budget) from the technical expertise of the PHS. Headquarters for the HCFA were maintained in Baltimore, away from other health offices with their headquarters in Washington. The administrative, budgetary, and physical separation of HCFA and the PHS was then complete. But whatever initial purpose it was meant to serve, this organization helped to complicate the AIDS effort.

Health Delivery Services

Health care planning, services, and education are the responsibility of the Health Resources and Services Administration (HRSA), a PHS agency that was created in 1982 as an umbrella for the Health Resources Administration (HRA), Health Services Administration (HSA), and the Office of Health Maintenance Organizations. The reorganization was an attempt to integrate the activities of the PHS with other public and private programs. According to official department literature, the HRA does health care planning, supports studies of the health care system and the training of health care professionals, and administers programs related to health care facilities, such as monitoring insured hospital construction loans. The HSA is concerned with inadequacies in the distribution of health care services and administers bureaus of community health services, medical services, health personnel development and service, and the Indian Health Service.

At first glance, the health planning, coordination, and educational roles seem ideally suited for response to a public health emergency. The HSA could, for example, make use of community health services for educating the community about disease transmission. But in 1981–1985 the groups being served by the HRSA (for example, American Indians in the Southwest) were initially so removed from groups at risk for AIDS that the agency's contributions were more theoretical and token than pragmatic.

In 1974, before the HRSA came into being, an attempt was made to coordinate the work of local and state health services through the National Health Planning and Resources Development Act.[8] Despite the explicit title of this legislation, its success is limited. It is even possible that it had an ironically opposite effect: the paperwork built into the act has slowed the ability of local authorities to administer their programs. In addition, the act was silent on the need for planning for emergency situations. Legislation specifically addressing health emergencies was not enacted until July 1983 as an amendment to the Public Health Service Act.

The Health Emergency Act had its origins in an earlier health crisis, Legionnaire's Disease, which broke out at the 1976 American Legion convention in Philadelphia. Richard Schweiker, then senator from Pennsylvania, conceived of an emergency fund for health research. His interest continued when he became secretary of HHS in 1981. Although the 1983 health emergency bill's origins were related to Legionnaire's Disease, health emergency funding became a truly political issue only with AIDS. The Health Emergency Act should have met the emergency patient care and management needs in AIDS but did not. Its aim was "To amend the Public Health Service Act to authorize appropriations to be made available to the Secretary of Health and Human Services for research for the cause, treatment and prevention of public health emergencies,"[9] but it lacked a plan for coordinating the health research establishment's response to emergency and had made no provisions for direct patient care and social services. Further, the original act did not clearly define when funds set aside for health emergency might be spent. Even when the bill was amended several years later to expand the fund to patient services, the coordination needs remained unmet. A comprehensive strategy for managing health emergencies still awaits development and application.

It would seem logical that all federal health institutions would be assessed for their potential contribution to an emergency effort. Yet the fragmented organization and often narrowly described missions of federal agencies may make such an assessment difficult. One example is the role of the VA, the government's largest independent agency and the nation's largest medical care system, with the primary purpose of providing direct patient services. In FY84, 32.7 percent of the

VA budget ($8.5 billion) was spent for hospital and medical care. That year approximately 84.6 million veterans and their dependents were potentially eligible for VA services.

Defining the VA's mission concerning AIDS relative to other health institutions was complicated because of the population believed to be at risk for the disease; that is, before 1985 some people doubted that AIDS could be spread from women to men. Consequently, the predominant ways of contracting AIDS among military personnel were thought to be homosexual behavior and IV drug abuse—behaviors which in 1985 carried military discharge and lack of VA responsibility for health care. With the understanding that AIDS is spread effectively by homosexual and heterosexual sex, and that both active and retired military personnel could require treatment, the VA's attention to this problem—and its coordination with other health institutions—becomes important. But despite the VA's presence in health research and care, the way to marshal the institution's resources during an essentially "nonmilitary" crisis has yet to be defined. Curiously, institutional linkages between the VA and PHS—which might have fostered early integration of AIDS activities—had existed earlier in the century. (The VA was established in 1930, having evolved from the PHS in 1922 as the Veterans Bureau.)[10]

Private organizations may also provide health services for specific communities, including those that are not eligible for standard health benefits. Moreover, nongovernment organizations could be in a better position to meet needs that the government may not be able or willing to address. A direct example can be found in AIDS, where public education was early seen as an important step in disease prevention. Educational materials would have to treat the issue of sexual behavior explicitly and directly.[11] Yet the subject of sex practices was a sensitive one, and the government was unwilling to prepare and distribute frank sexual literature. The practical question of whose responsibility it is to provide such information remains an unresolved question that continues to thwart effective public education.

In 1984 the CDC's Center for Professional Development and Training conducted a nine-city survey to assess collaborative efforts between the public health providers and the community organizations working toward AIDS prevention through education. In a preliminary April 1985 report, the CDC workers stressed the importance of close cooperation between the public health providers and the community organizations, pointing out that the latter were essential as bridges between the public health services and the at-risk groups, which were generally isolated from mainstream society. In the AIDS health emergency, newly formed private organizations have played a significant role in public education, delivery of medical and support services, and in supporting research initiatives. Yet the traditional foundation world has been late to the party. According to the Council on Foundations, only five of the nation's leading philanthropies financed the AIDS-related programs.[12] The largest foundation initiative—the Robert Wood Johnson Foundation's $17.2-million effort to support community-based and home care—did not make its first grant until 1987.

Organizational Problems of Coordinating a Health Emergency

Most federal resources available for response to public health emergencies such as polio and AIDS have been located within a single department of the executive branch of government since the late 1930s. But the independent origins and operations of the different agencies as well as their size and division of responsibilities turn the task of coordinating them into an enormous job. The task is complicated by a legacy of institutional reorganizations undertaken in response to changing views about health care and the appropriate role of government over the past two hundred years.

The separation of the PHS agencies from other HHS components is central to understanding the federal response to a health emergency. Federal successes and failures in AIDS stemmed from the strict definition of the AIDS problem as a

PHS issue, when necessary activities fell under the authority of HCFA, a separate branch of the same department. Former Assistant Secretary for Health Brandt has often commented that during the first years of the AIDS epidemic, "PHS may have had only 3 percent of the HHS budget, but it had the majority of the problem!" Yet issues of payment for health care delivery, experimental therapies, and clinical research were fast becoming of central importance, although their federal oversight lay in large part outside the PHS.

This problem, acute in the AIDS crisis, was characteristic of federal oversight of health. It was recognized early in the Reagan administration and was noted in the February 1981 White House press release announcing the new PHS head. A further attempt to redress the HHS organizational problem took the form of a bill that was introduced but not enacted in the 98th Congress to merge the management of PHS and HCFA under a single undersecretary for Health and Human Services.[13]

As the AIDS epidemic entered its sixth year, discussion continued over the issue of who should be in charge. One suggestion, attributed to Dr. James Mason, then acting assistant secretary for health, was that the surgeon general might play a coordinating role.[14] But even when the surgeon general did begin to speak about AIDS, it was as a public health spokesman, and not as a coordinator with any authority. As the issue remained unresolved for AIDS, it also remained unresolved for future emergency efforts.

Thus the AIDS experience forced attention to four general areas that characterize the delivery of health care services in the 1980s. Common to each was the need to define clearly the roles of federal, state, and local authorities as well as the roles of different health professionals. First was the role of the primary care physician in the emergency effort, especially as this related to the clinical research effort. Second was the problem of how experimental therapy would be funded and administered. Third was the problem of funding and providing public education and psychosocial services. Fourth was the issue of funding and providing a consistent level of health care services across the country.

5

Economics and Politics

I N 1984 Americans spent $387.4 billion on health—about 10 percent of the gross national product.[1] National health expenditures were borne 56 percent by consumers, 41 percent by the government, and 3 percent by philanthropy and industry. And of the $160.3 billion spent from public coffers, 70 percent came from the federal treasury. Thus only about 30 percent of national health expenditures came from federal tax revenues. Tax payments support three sectors of the health care establishment, but disproportionately. Virtually all public health surveillance and monitoring is supported by government (federal and local) funds. Federal funds also support the greater part of the basic biomedical research establishment, with the remainder funded by private and nonprofit sources. So although nearly 80 percent of federal health outlays in 1984 went to health care services (including Medicaid), the national bill for health services and supplies received 61 percent of its support from nongovernment sources. Even when government funds are not specifically earmarked for a health-related program, however, the direction of that program is shaped by the national health policy as expressed in the federal budget.

The Federal Budget as a Political Statement

Every January, within fifteen days after Congress convenes, the president submits his budget for the coming fiscal year. Published by the Government Printing Office in a distinctive paperback edition, the president's budget is a guaranteed best seller. Those interested in the direction of the administration's policy anxiously await its publication. Yet, although eagerly anticipated, the budget is never a complete surprise. It is the culmination of almost three years of work, and it is just the start of negotiations between the administration and the Congress. When the process works according to schedule, these negotiations result in the adoption of a budget resolution before the fiscal year begins on October 1.

The final budget resolution is a patchwork compromise of the views of all who participate in the budget process—the different parts of government, the press, the public policy community (think tanks, commentators, former officials), and lobbyists representing a multitude of interests. The final budget's form reflects the deals cut within the executive branch, among the congressional representatives of diverse constituencies, and between the Congress and the administration. Rarely do the January budget and the final resolution match. To understand the budget process is therefore to understand that the economics and politics of any federal effort are inextricably entwined, for the budget is fundamentally a political statement.

The federal budget reflects the culmination of two different but simultaneous exercises. In a structured ritual, the administration's policy is first set out in the president's budget. The Congress responds by a presentation of its budget. The president has the opportunity to veto the Congress's package and, in turn, the Congress can override a presidential veto. Economic analysis to support the executive and congressional branches' efforts is provided by the Office of Management and Budget (OMB) and the Congressional Budget Office (CBO).[2] The federal budget process results in a blueprint of all federal activities for a fiscal year. The steps of this highly iterative and confusing process, which was at work during the first five years of the AIDS epidemic, are laid out in the budget acts of 1921 and 1973.[3] The sequence of the various steps is instructive, as it indicates the myriad points for political influence and intervention.

The President's Budget

The presidential budget cycle begins in early March, when federal agencies submit to the OMB their preliminary budget reviews. Starting agency budgets are based on the budget projections submitted in previous years. Independently, the OMB, the Council of Economic Advisors (CEA), and the Treasury Department make projections on the economic outlook and estimated revenue levels.

Throughout the spring, the OMB holds discussions with the agency staffs, and by June the OMB director advises the president about the agencies' preliminary plans. The president makes tentative budget policy decisions on total outlays, receipts, and major program issues. Guidelines reflecting these decisions are communicated by the OMB to the agencies in the form of planning targets. In October and November the OMB receives and reviews formal submissions, and each agency or department presents and defends its programs. By the end of November the OMB director prepares budget recommendations for the president.

During the month of December—after the president's review of the budget—program decisions and approved allowances are transmitted to each agency head, who may accept these decisions, appeal to OMB, or even appeal directly to the president. At the same time, final projections about the economic outlook and prospective revenues are made. Together with emerging outlay estimates, OMB, CEA, and the Treasury Department recommend last-minute changes that will affect the size of the budget surplus or deficit. Within fifteen days after Congress convenes for the new year, the president relays his Budget Document and Message to Congress.

The Congressional Budget

While the presidential budget is nearing completion, the congressional cycle just begins. The process starts by November 10, when the president submits the Current Services budget to Congress detailing the cost of continuing the authorized, existing programs from the previous fiscal year into the new fiscal year without policy change (that is, without program expansions or contractions). The document also makes assumptions about inflation, unemployment, and the real rate of economic growth. By December 31 the Joint Economic Committee (composed of members of the Senate and House), having reviewed the Current Services budget, reports its findings to Congress. In late January the Congressional Budget Office (CBO) submits forecasts for the one-year and five-year economic outlook and estimates of the baseline (Current Services) budget to the president.

In February and through March, with the president's budget in hand, the House and Senate Budget Committees hold hearings and begin drafting budget legislation. This legislation authorizes an agency to carry out a specific program, but it does not provide funding. The actual appropriation of dollars for a program is a separate, and usually subsequent act.

On March 15, all committees and joint committees submit to the Budget Committees estimates and views on the federal government's outlays and budget authority for the ensuing fiscal year. A month later the House and Senate Budget Committees draw up, reconcile, and report a tentative First Concurrent Resolution that sets target totals for budget authority, outlays, receipts, and the public debt, and guides subsequent consideration of appropriations and tax measures to their respective houses. Because budget resolutions in each house usually differ, and because both houses need to establish identical resolutions, time is needed to work out the differences. This occurs through House-Senate conference. A concurrent resolution must be adopted by May 15; Congress then begins consideration of appropriations and other bills to allow new spending effective in the next fiscal year.

The House Appropriations Committee holds hearings and debates on requests on the floor of the House. Next, the appropriations and tax bills are forwarded to the Senate where a similar process occurs. Differences between the houses on appropriation bills are again reconciled in Conference Committee, with the resulting legislation transmitted to the president for his approval or veto. All appropriations bills must be passed by the seventh day after Labor Day, and by September 15 a Second Concurrent Resolution is passed.

If separate congressional decisions taken during the appropriations process are not consistent with the second concurrent budget totals, the resolution may ask for changes. The House and Senate Budget Committees then combine these changes and report them in a Reconciliation Bill. By September 25 Congress formally completes the budget process by enacting the Second Concurrent Resolution. After this point Congress may not consider any spending or revenue legislation that would alter budget figures from those specified in the Second Resolution. On October 1 the fiscal year begins.

There is still room for change after the budget is adopted. If the need arises, Congress may adopt a new budget resolution during the fiscal year. Departments may request supplemental appropriations, and can also request a different allocation of funds through a budget amendment. Frequently, budget amendments are requested retrospectively. The Congress can also provide supplemental funds, even when the administration finds them to be unnecessary. These mechanisms, however, may be insufficient to meet the needs of a health emergency. The problems have been expressed in the public debate over funding for AIDS as "the nation's number one priority." The question most asked during congressional hearings concerning AIDS was: How could AIDS be the nation's number one priority if it receives so little funding? The question persisted although, at least during the earliest part of the epidemic, funding was not the most important issue. But because politics and money are inseparable in Washington, the focus was appropriate.

Because of the formal rules of the budget process and the urgency of an emergency, the first response to an emergency happens when budgeted funds are diverted, and documented only retrospectively. Although such reallocations have often been made, resorting to them emphasizes the unique requirements of managing a health emergency—flexibility to respond decisively in a way that builds confidence in the federal establishment's leadership. Instead, the most frequent real result of this procedure is friction, arising when pragmatic emergency needs are frustrated by the normal system. In one exchange between PHS officials and an oversight committee on how the budget for AIDS was developed in the early period, HHS Assistant Secretary Edward Brandt explained his position: in an emergency, funds are taken from another program, or Congress is asked to provide supplemental funds. "That is the way the Congress has asked us to behave. That is what we do."[4]

Disbursing Money for Health Care

The choice, amount, and distribution of federal funding for health care activities vary in response to the prevailing political ideology, public opinion, and the state of the economy. For example, in the 1930s, the distribution of health care responsibilities was impaired by the Great Depression, and "The responsibilities for performing local public health services (and many other social services such as education) continued to rest with the states, which delegated them to the cities and localities, but the base for tax collection was steadily moving from the localities and states to the federal level."[5]

In response to the political and economic realities of the 1930s, the Social Security Act of 1935 established grants-in-aid for health; these were intended to provide some equity in the available resources for health care and to establish uniform standards of health care services and delivery across the nation. Fifty years later, the dominant political philosophy had shifted. Popular enthusiasm moved Washington to return the responsibility for an increasing number of social programs, as well as the tax base which supported these services, back to the states. This was in no small part a response to the recession of the 1980s. The differing dominant political philosophies of the 1930s, the 1960s, and 1980s were reflected in how health programs were financed.

The instruments for federal support of health fall into three categories: block grants, categorical program grants, and individual program grants. Title VI of the Social Security Act and later the Public Health Service Act provide guidance for the criteria to be used in establishing formulas for distribution of federal revenues to the states. These criteria include consideration of a state's population, its economic status, and the prevalence of public health programs.

The general-purpose block grants are distributed to the states by formula and have little restriction on how the states spend the funds. In general, the majority of these funds are distributed by state governments to local health departments. The Reagan administration has preferred block grants because they allow the greatest amount of local discretion concerning how federal funds are spent.

Categorical program grants are also distributed to the states by formula, but include specific program restrictions on expenditure categories. Some funds are distributed to local health authorities. Individual project grants, the third category, are awarded to applicants directly and generally bypass the state bureaucracy. Applicants may be either individuals or institutions (governmental and nongovernmental).

It is evident that the type of funding will determine how closely the federal establishment controls local health programs. Thus block grants place discretion for health policy with state government, whereas individual grants can sever a state government's influence from local programs. Predominant use of categorical grants provides the greatest leverage for federal domination of health policy at the state and local levels.

Sometimes federal policy concerning local delivery of health services is determined by the availability of funding instruments. In the early period of AIDS federal resources were absent. In the course of congressional testimony concerning who paid for locally delivered services in the initial period of the AIDS epidemic, Congresswoman Barbara Boxer (D-California) asked San Francisco's Director of Public Health Mervyn Silverman for an estimate of the proportion of federal funds available to the San Francisco AIDS efforts.[6] Silverman replied: "We have at this time [summer of 1983] at least one representative from CDC helping us with our epidemiologic investigations. If you eliminate that, you eliminate pretty much the federal input . . . For our problems, it is probably 98-plus percent local funds."

Silverman's comments confirmed what a report from the Council of Mayors was later to document—that the lion's share of locally delivered services in AIDS education, counseling, and so on, occurred without federal guidance and funding.

In answer to the same question about federal funds, the New York City Health Commissioner David Sencer said: "not talking about hospitals or diagnostic services, about 25 per cent [of funding] may come from the federal assistance . . . It is the one opportunity we have had to use the block grant."

Local health officials thus pick up the largest part of the bill for delivering social services during a public health emergency, and the items on the bill may well vary from locality to locality. These items are not the only variables: a "locality" may be a city or a county. Moreover, the amount of the public health bill that can be paid from federal funds made available to local officials will vary with the particular services needed and the relation between a locality and its state. Sencer's comment referred to the fact that federal block grant funds for sexually transmitted diseases were used in New York City for the AIDS effort.[7]

The debate on Capitol Hill concerning payment for AIDS-related activities was on one level the continuation of a discussion that has been taking place since the late 1700s—the definition of the roles that the federal, state, and local authorities were to play in the payment and delivery of health services. This perennial problem was further complicated by the budgetary difficulties of financing a health emergency, and by the highly localized nature of the AIDS epidemic. For example, Mervyn Silverman has often said: "If I lived west of the Mississippi and were diagnosed with AIDS, I would crawl to San Francisco"[8]—a comment on the absence of AIDS services in many cities and the concentration of expertise in a few urban areas.

Ironically, the cities with the health emergency knowhow developed a political and fiscal problem on that account. Although health services were locally managed and financed, their patients came from broader geographical regions. In San Francisco in 1985, conservative estimates were that at least 15 percent of the AIDS patients were not local residents and had come to that city only for medical treatment. The resulting burden was not easily met, nor envisioned, in the formulas used to dispense federal funds. Thus the AIDS emergency continually reiterated the need to revisit the historic conflicts between local control of health service delivery and centralized federal activities to see if (and how) the roles of federal, state, and local health authorities—including fiscal support—should be altered during a public health emergency.

Points of Political Influence

Throughout the budget process the opinions and influence of players in the public policy process can have an effect at numerous points. These pressure points are different for the presidential and congressional budgets, because the extent to which the budget debate is conducted in public also differs.

The presidential process is essentially conducted "behind closed doors." In fact, in addressing the question "was enough spent on AIDS," much of the argument between PHS officials and congressional oversight committees focused on how the administration's budget was constructed. But OMB policy often barred such disclosures: "Historically, the executive branch communications that have led to the preparation of the budget have not been disclosed by the agencies or by those who have prepared the budget."[9]

The points least understood by the public and of greatest sensitivity in the formulation of the president's budget are therefore negotiations between OMB and the executive branch agencies. OMB's power lies in its intermediary role. Critics of any federal health response are often drawn to find the cause in the HHS-OMB interaction. For example, Phil Lee, director of the Institute for Health Policy at the University of California at San Francisco, and a former HEW assistant secretary for health in the Johnson administration, has stated the belief that too limited funds for federal AIDS activities reflected policy at the OMB.[10]

In contrast to the presidential budget, at least a portion of the congressional budget process occurs in public. The numerous congressional committees have diverse roles and power. The most prestigious, because of their direct effect on the budget, are the House and Senate budget committees and the individual authorization and appropriation committees. Other committees also have real power, largely because their activities influence the decisions of the budget committees.

With health emergency funding, it is important to emphasize that it is easier to trace direct financing of public health monitoring and basic research than payment for health care and social services. The ease of retrospective accounting—a byproduct of the budget process—mirrors the fragmented and pluralistic nature of health care delivery. Further, because AIDS was initially defined as a research problem, federal outlays have been predominantly tied to PHS efforts.

In examining the finances for AIDS as a case study of whether the ordinary budget process can accommodate a health emergency, it must be remembered that the start of the epidemic coincided with a time when the overriding federal budgetary concern was a reduction of the federal deficit, to be achieved by reducing spending for domestic programs. The AIDS budget therefore has to be understood as a compromise between responding to the epidemic without emasculating other necessary health programs and heading the political imperative to decrease federal government spending.

The first appearance of an AIDS item in the PHS budget can be traced to FY82. Therefore any outlays that were made between the anecdotal reports in 1979, the *Morbidity and Mortality Weekly Report* (*MMWR*) case findings in 1981, and the more mature understanding of the epidemic in early 1982 were the result of reallocation decisions. According to the HHS, the total amount in millions the PHS expended for AIDS in FY82 was $5.5, increased to $28.7 in FY83, $61.4 in FY84 and $108.6 in FY85.[11] AIDS expenditures are estimated as $233.7 for FY86, $410.7 for FY87 and $433.6 for FY88. A reasoned opinion on whether these increasing expenditures fulfill the needs of the AIDS emergency—as well as an understanding of how the figures were developed—must consider details of the budget process, be sensitive to the differences between budget authorizations and budget appropriations, and take into account how allocated funds direct the activities of the health care delivery, research, and public monitoring institutions (see Tables 2, 3, and 4).

The Lesson of Gramm-Rudman-Hollings

An embellishment to the federal budget process was added in 1985. The Balanced Budget and Emergency Deficit Control Act of 1985—otherwise known by the names of its sponsors, senators Gramm, Rudman, and Hollings—was passed by the Congress at the end of the December session of the 98th Congress and took effect in January 1986. The bill required automatic, across-the-board spending cuts to achieve a schedule of federal deficit reductions between 1986 and 1991. A 4.3 percent cut was mandated for all nonexempted federal programs in FY86. Although a key part of Gramm-Rudman-Hollings was eventually found to be unconstitutional, how the AIDS budget was handled under the terms of the legislation is relevant in assessing the wisdom of linking emergency and annual budgets.

Few federal programs were exempt from the budget-cutting legislation, including those that were earmarked for the AIDS health emergency effort. But the public debate about Gramm-Rudman-Hollings and AIDS research was indistinguishable from the discussion about any domestic program. Debate centered not on whether enough research was planned and funded, but on whether the now adequate AIDS research program could sustain the automatic cuts of Gramm-Rudman-

Table 2.   Public Health Service Funding for AIDS (in millions)

	1982 Act.[a]	1983 Act.	1984 Act.	1985 Act.	1986 Est.[b]	1987 Est.	1988 Est.
HRSA	0	0	0	0	0	1.9	6.6
CDC	2.0	6.2	13.7	33.2	55.2[c]	89.0	112.0
NIH							
NCI	2.40	9.80	16.62	26.87	45.05	61.7	—
NHLBI	.005	1.20	4.87	9.32	15.47	17.1	—
NIDR	.02	.02	.08	.09	1.71	2.7	—
NINCDS	.03	.07	1.51	1.16	1.43	2.2	—
NIAID	.30	9.22	19.61	23.27	63.28	145.8	—
NICHD	0	0	0	0	1.40	2.2	—
NEI	.03	.04	.06	.20	.09	.1	—
DRR	.56	.70	1.35	2.80	6.15	6.1	—
OD	0	0	0	0	.07	10.0	—
Subtotal NIH	3.3	21.6	44.1	63.7	141.5[c]	247.9	343.5
ADAMHA							
NIMH	0	.20	1.20	1.90	5.05	13.8	—
NIDA	0	.31	1.58	.67	7.10	31.3	—
NIAAA	0	0	0	0	0	2.3	—
Subtotal ADAMHA	0	.51	2.79	2.57	12.15	47.5	55.0
AIDS Coordinator	0	0	0	0	0	0	—
OASH	0	0	0	0	0	0	0.8
Gen. Dept. Management	0	0	0	0	15.3	10.0	—
FDA	.1	.3	.8	9.0	9.5	14.3	15.7
TOTAL[d]	5.4	28.06	61.4	118.44	233.7	410.5	553.6

[a] Actual dollars spent.
[b] Estimated dollars.
[c] 6.9 million was transferred from CDC to NIH for drug intervention.
[d] Including some expenditures not itemized above.
Source: AIDS Action Council, Washington, D.C. (January 1987).

Table 3. Federal AIDS Funding during the Initial Period (in thousands of dollars)

Fiscal year	PHS request	President's request	Congressional appropriation
1982	0	0	5,555
1983	—	0	28,736
1984	59,903	39,827	61,460
1985	91,051	60,589	108,618

Source: Office of Technology Assessment, *National Journal* (August 30, 1986).

Hollings. Hence this discussion marked a change from the public perception of AIDS as an acute, extraordinary emergency in the initial period to a perception of AIDS as a chronic public health concern. Moreover, the automatic cuts mandated in this legislation limited budgetary flexibility even more thoroughly than before, whereas the hallmark of emergency management is the ability to change direction quickly. The lesson of Gramm-Rudman-Hollings, therefore, was that in the midst of a health emergency the response continued to be tied to the increasingly inflexible annual budget.

This conclusion is not limited to research funds alone. For example, it was only in FY86 that the legislators recognized the need for direct federal assistance to heavily affected cities and allocated $16 million to four experimental treatment centers in

Table 4. PHS AIDS Disbursements during the Initial Period (in percentages)

Agency	FY82	FY83	FY84	FY85
NIH	60.40	75.54	71.79	63.75
FDA	2.70	1.22	1.30	9.18
CDC	36.90	21.62	22.37	24.14
ADAMHA	—	1.62	4.54	2.93
TOTAL	100.00	100.00	100.00	100.00

Source: Health and Human Services, National Institutes of Health, Office of Technology Assessment, 1985 Report, "Federal Response to AIDS."

areas with a high incidence of the disease.[12] Yet by January 1986 the $16 million was in jeopardy. Although appropriated in the fall of the previous year, the money still had not been committed by the end of it because of a political hold on spending federal funds to distribute literature that some viewed as being porno-graphic. At the same time, the Gramm-Rudman-Hollings leg-islation imposed a pragmatic goal for HHS to cut spending. Because the money had not been committed, HHS decided to cut the $16 million even beyond Gramm-Rudman-Hollings. The argument was that it is easier to return uncommitted money to the Treasury than to cut an ongoing program. The sum was a drop in the bucket of the overall PHS budget, but it was symbolic of a year's fight to have federal relief for locally funded AIDS health services. Not surprisingly, the congressional staff that had worked to authorize the funds six months earlier began to prepare for hearings to lambast the cut. Asked about whether the hearings would be held before or after the March 1 deadline mandated by the then active rules of Gramm-Rudman-Hollings to announce deficit reduction decisions, one congres-sional staffer said, "If the hearings are held before the announcement, we will embarrass the administration into changing the policy. Alternatively, we will thrash them for making the decision."[13] The effect on the AIDS budget of the Gramm-Rudman-Hollings bill illustrates how the line item approach to budgeting impedes flexibility in managing an emergency response.

6

Unique Elements of a Health Emergency

T HE CATCHY phrase "the nation's number one health priority" that Edward Brandt had used to emphasize the seriousness with which the government viewed the AIDS crisis was to reappear in other contexts. Laurence Miike and Denise Dougherty, of the Office of Technology Assessment (OTA), conducted interviews in September 1984 that became the basis of an OTA report on "both the technical aspects of research and related issues of public health policy"[1] of the AIDS emergency. When the report appeared in February 1985, the conclusions emphasized a disjunction between the amount of funding and the labeling of AIDS as the nation's number one health priority. Press reviews described the report as critical and even condemnatory of the national health effort.

Responding to this criticism, the PHS held that the OTA report was self-contradictory, praising the rapid scientific advances that had been made while faulting the health service for inadequate funding of the research effort. From a distance, the disagreement may have simply reflected the frustration of all who engaged in the AIDS effort—the disease was eluding control despite dramatic scientific advances. Yet the OTA touched on problems basic to health emergency management, among them personnel reallocation, assignment of fiscal responsibility in the separate components of HHS, and lack of discretion for rebudgeting across bureaucratic lines. Each of these problems showed how the normal, politically negotiated budget process fails to meet crises.

It is hard to imagine that any one time is convenient for a health emergency to occur, but the early 1980s were clearly ill suited for it. Faced with inflation and unemployment, a conservative administration began to cut domestic spending. The swing to fiscal conservatism was accompanied by a move to transfer the authority and the revenue base for many programs from the federal government to the states. The new management at OMB mandated overall government retrenchment, with the result that CDC and FDA lost 25 to 30 percent in operational costs, capital expenditures, and personnel. In FY82, CDC alone reduced its personnel approximately 30 percent. Curiously, when critics of the government's efforts found the agency's early response to the AIDS crisis to be inadequate, the mandated cuts were erroneously interpreted as being "AIDS specific" and, by some, as revealing an ideological, anti-AIDS conspiracy within the administration.[2] In fact, the budget cuts predated the epidemic.

Any consideration of how resources can be tapped for an emergency requires a look at reallocation policies, congressionally initiated supplemental appropriation requests, and the use of emergency funds. With the consent of OMB and Congress, dollars can be moved between budget categories within the PHS. During the first three and a half years of the AIDS crisis, all AIDS programs were funded solely from PHS sources, without any rebudgeting from other HHS programs. No supplemental appropriations were formally requested from Congress by the administration, although additional funds were earmarked for AIDS through congressionally initiated supplemental appropriations. Thus HHS seemed to have effectively developed a "covert" means for obtaining additional funds without using formal channels—a development that is instructive in clarifying the distinction between the appropriations and authorizations processes and in exemplifying how congressional turf battles (sometimes on the same side of the aisle) can impede an emergency response.

On May 9, 1983, Henry Waxman's congressional subcommittee held hearings on the Public Health Emergency Act. The act proposed to establish a $40 million standing contingency fund "to authorize appropriations to be made available to the Secretary of Health and Human Services for research for the cause, treatment and prevention of public health emergencies."[3] In presenting the administration's attitude, Edward Brandt testified:

We believe that this legislation is unnecessary; that we have ample authority now to take all the actions necessary to deal with public health emergencies, both through research grants and contracts, through other PHS activities, such as investigations and recall of products . . .

We are strongly committed to a vigorous research program for AIDS and other diseases that create public health emergencies, and to a quick, direct response in all other ways necessary to the public health. While we disagree with the specific technical mechanism proposed in this bill, we welcome the subcommittee's attention to this question.[4]

Waxman then questioned the inconsistency:

I find your testimony very peculiar in light of the fact that just two years ago Secretary Schweiker came in and proposed this very idea of a public health emergency response fund . . .

Now the administration's position, despite the Secretary's request two years ago, is that you don't need it. What did the administration think was necessary when they requested the idea of this fund originally and what has happened to change the administration's mind?[5]

Brandt recalled that he argued this position because politically he had no alternative, with the PHS caught in a power struggle between congressional authorizations and appropriations committees. The authorizations committees set the ground rules and maximum levels for funding—but it is the appropriations committee that actually dispenses the funds. The health emergency act proposed to establish a standing fund through the House Energy and Commerce Committee, which has an authorizing role. The appropriations committee, chaired by William H. Natcher (D-Kentucky), argued that such a standing fund should not be established by an authorizing committee. At stake was a potential shift in power, and Brandt understood that he could not afford to get on the "bad side" of the appropriations committee.

This interpretation is reinforced by the resolution of a similar question concerning a contingency fund for emergency needs at the FDA. House oversight for authorizing the NIH, CDC, and FDA programs resided with Waxman's subcommittee, but appropriations for FDA were handled by a House committee other than those for NIH and CDC. All the while that the administration was opposing H.R. 2713 (the health emergency act), in the light of off-the-record conversations held between Natcher and Brandt, an FDA contingency fund was approved. Brandt, in responding to Waxman's query, tried to articulate the political reality: "We have not changed our view. We are, however, attempting to live within the appropriation committee's direction."[6]

Following the identification of a viral etiology for AIDS in the spring of 1984, Brandt found another way to seek funds, which appeared to circumvent established budget policy. He established and chaired an executive committee of PHS heads involved in the AIDS effort[7] and requested that the committee assess, first, what AIDS-related programs could be phased out and the amount of money saved; and second, what new programs would be needed to exploit the discoveries of the AIDS virus. Brandt then offered these recommendations in a memorandum to HHS secretary Margaret Heckler in support of his request for supplemental funds.[8]

It is a common assumption in the bureaucracy that once words are on paper, they are at high risk for distribution; the memo that Brandt sent to Heckler was leaked and was subsequently to achieve notoriety as an example of how PHS officials got around the administration's policy not to ask for new monies. Virginia Apuzzo, then Executive Director of the National Gay and Lesbian Taskforce, recalls, for example, that a copy of that memo came addressed to her through the mails in a plain brown wrapper.[9] Brandt categorically denies any knowledge of how the memo was leaked, although he notes that no special or unusual precautions were taken to prevent such a leak. At the same time he readily acknowledges why it was written—to argue with OMB for more funds. Thus although the memo was never formally transmitted to Congress and the administration never formally requested the funds the memo described, the needs of the PHS were in fact expressed to the Congress and once again, supplemental monies were provided.

Even in 1985, when the publicity that accompanied Rock Hudson's death forced a public outcry for more AIDS research, HHS persisted in not requesting supplemental funds. Nevertheless the funds were forthcoming, and less than three months after Hudson's death $234.2 million was mandated for FY86 AIDS effort. Following the pattern that had earlier been established, funds were made available without the administration's ever breaking its policy pledge to cut domestic spending.

Any reasonable analysis of how AIDS was financed recognizes that the PHS was trapped in political and financial circumstances that did not allow economic flexibility at the departmental level. On the other side, there is a little to suggest that the lack of OMB enthusiasm for supplemental requests reflected a specific anti-AIDS posture. Rather, the PHS could spend as it liked on AIDS so long as they took the funds from their own or other, nameless coffers. However, it is also likely that politically sensitive officials in the PHS recognized that a more vocal anti-AIDS stand could evoke a reaction from the radical right that could cause difficulties for the PHS, as the White House might then be obliged to become directly involved. Ironically, the more militant anti-AIDS groups in the homosexual community saw the lack of presidential comment early in the AIDS crisis as a deficit. More likely the silence from the White House helped the PHS get on with its real business. (Few remembered that during the 1976 swine flu scare, direct intervention of President Ford forced the development of a policy that PHS officials found to complicate rather than expedite orderly public health measures.)[10]

Throughout 1986, the OMB continued to maintain the position that it was unwilling to rebudget across agencies for the health emergency. Anger at this attitude was in part based on a popular misconception—especially mistaken at a time when the Congress was committed to deficit reduction—that funds cut from one program become available for others. The popular argument that there would be more funds for AIDS research if the defense budget were decreased was fallacious. The money cut out was supposed to decrease the national deficit; it would not become available for other uses. In essence, it vanished.

Funding Basic Research

The report eventually released by Ted Weiss's oversight sub-committee on the efforts of HHS in the AIDS crisis concluded that the funding of AIDS research in the extramural community by NIH had been "unnecessarily delayed." Because of this delay, other research efforts had to be redirected for work on AIDS. The second main criticism was directed at the inability of the NIH grants and contracts system to provide rapid funding of urgent problems.[11] The report also implied that reallocating resources was detrimental to the initial AIDS effort. In this the committee showed that it had not grasped the concept that any early emergency effort is by definition a reallocation exercise—the initial detective work done by CDC epidemiologists and NIH researchers was supported through the reshuffling of resources. The appropriate concern is how to reallocate with minimal disruption to other research efforts, and to determine whether reallocation is equally sensible in intramural and extramural programs.

The ability of NIH to redirect its resources during an emergency is limited by three factors. First, although the NIH budget is negotiated annually, most programs span several years; therefore more than 85 percent of any year's budget has already been committed, restricting both ordinary budgeting and reallocation. Second, approximately 80 percent of the NIH research budget is committed to extramural programs, which are conducted at nonfederal facilities. Third, NIH operations in general—and responsibility for its research priorities in particular—are highly decentralized within the agency.

An effective initial response to a health emergency must be

rapid, avoid duplicating research, and be able to draw on the collective advice and guidance of both the intramural and extramural scientific community. There has been little disagreement that intramural scientists responded quickly to the AIDS challenge. The question is how efficiently they identified and focused on the research. The next step is to examine whether the internal emphasis could have changed as information expanded, or whether, once the "turf" was established, it was difficult to give up.

The work of Robert Gallo's laboratory at the National Cancer Institute is generally used as evidence that the intramural programs at NIH responded quickly to the AIDS challenge. AIDS-related activities at NIH were concentrated in three institutes: the National Heart, Lung, and Blood Institute (NHLBI), the National Institute for Allergy and Infectious Diseases (NIAID), and the National Cancer Institute (NCI). NHLBI coordinated efforts to ensure a safe blood supply through its participation in the national blood program. NIAID made initial attempts to identify the infectious agent and to understand the immune deficiency. In the second period NIAID concentrated on antiviral therapeutics and immune reconstitution. NCI's involvement is the least obvious and most curious. It illustrates the nature of historic accident in establishing scientific turf and the frequency with which initial research successes reflect the strength of fundamental research programs that predate the crisis.

The rise in cases of the rare Kaposi's sarcoma sparked the interest of NCI in the possibility of a cancer epidemic. When the tumor was understood to be neither the primary nor the lethal manifestation, one might have logically expected NCI's interest in AIDS to diminish. However, the retroviral nature of the AIDS virus assured that NCI would remain interested, for its scientists had been actively studying retroviruses because of their tumor-inducing properties. Since the early 1970s the Special Virus Cancer Program mandated by the National Cancer Act focused on the basic biology of these viruses. A large and sophisticated retroviral research capability existed both in the intramural and extramural

NCI programs and was directed—first in small part, later in large part—toward AIDS. The ability to mount a vigorous, AIDS-specific retroviral research program is therefore directly traced to the background of decades of basic cancer research.

Once the AIDS virus had been identified and the efforts at NIH shifted to a hunt for antiviral drugs and prevention, the research effort was divided. A $140 million supplement allocated in the fall of 1985 was placed in the NIH director's office. Eventually this sum was to be divided evenly between NCI and NIAID, with the director seemingly maintaining only token oversight of the effort—a decentralized way of doing things at NIH, where only infrequently has central NIH management appeared to dominate program direction. The distribution of AIDS funds hinted that the central administration was interested in maintaining parity between two potentially rival institutes, rather than dividing the money on the basis of the individual strengths of the two institutes.

Public attention has focused more on NIH's extramural AIDS research policy than on its intramural programs, and specifically on whether enough was done to mobilize scientists who were ordinarily supported through the RO1 (investigator-initiated) grant mechanism. In the decade preceding the AIDS epidemic, a smaller and smaller proportion of such grant proposals was actually getting funded. A question to ask in general about U.S. biomedical research was whether enough sound scientific proposals (as measured by a peer-review study section's approval) were funded (where the pay line is set). The next concern was whether AIDS-related research was and should have been assigned "lower" pay lines in view of the public health emergency nature of AIDS, and whether enough AIDS research was funded as early as possible. The debate reveals a general presumption that the more dollars are spent, the faster results are achieved. In fact there is no one-to-one relation between dollars expended and useful results.

If the general agreement is that intramural programs responded quickly but that extramural efforts lagged, what would have been an appropriate time for extramural scientific effort to become involved? According to the Weiss and OTA reports, extramural scientists might have redirected their efforts to work on AIDS, which would have been contrary to the terms of their grants. In American biomedical science, initial experiments in a new field historically have used resources solicited for other purposes. But how to get new funds for new purposes quickly, in the midst of a crisis? Even in noncrisis times, the need for preliminary data to solicit support for future work is a well known problem. The White House Science Council panel, convened to study the health of academic science, recommended a shift to awards from three to five years and suggested that investigators be allowed to use up to 10 percent of their funds on a discretionary basis to support activities not necessarily covered by the grant.[12]

In examining how research related to novel health emergencies can be initiated, the issue is not how the ordinary extramural program processes can be hastened. What is needed is a mechanism that does not now exist—and cannot be designed until the roles of intramural and extramural scientists in a crisis effort are clearly defined. These roles may well be difficult for the extramural scientist to accept, because dependence on government decision is counter to a scientific culture that shuns coordination and encourages the slow development of peer consensus. Assigning research responsibilities is almost as foreign and "anti-American" to the science community at large as is, to the public at large, the concept that the solution to a problem will require more than just more money.

Coordination of Efforts

Because no cure or vaccine was quickly found for AIDS, questions persist about the lack of coordination in the scientific research community as a possible reason for lack of progress.

Arthur S. Levine's office headed the initial strategic AIDS research planning efforts for the National Cancer Institute. Reflecting on the federal response in 1983, Dr. Levine concluded:

It becomes important to distinguish science from government . . . The intramural programs of the NIH and the CDC responded instantaneously to the epidemic of AIDS and the need for research, both epidemiologic as well as virologic and immunologic, as soon as the intellectual ideas jelled—there had to be some time for people to have a sense of what was going on. As soon as they had performed that feat of intellection, work started. And it started through normal mechanisms; there was no need to pass new legislation. No need to lobby. No need to have peer review. There was a good and vast federal mechanism for immediately responding. I think the response—in retrospect—was, at least for NIH and CDC, astonishingly rapid.[13]

Is the criticism that the establishment failed to act with dispatch valid, or is it simply an expression of frustration? Other critics of the federal response to AIDS have suggested that the reason for the lack of progress was not so much lack of coordination as lack of interest; that scientists initially stayed away from AIDS because it was primarily a disease of homosexual men.

Although this perception is difficult to document, NIH and CDC scientists who initially participated in organizing AIDS research efforts noted a tendency among fellow scientists either to discount or to deny the seriousness of the disease. How much of this reaction should be attributed to fear or ignorance is unclear. In the opinion of James Curran, who headed the CDC's AIDS efforts, scientists avoided issues that relate to sex and had little understanding of homosexuality or of the epidemiology of a disease such as AIDS. He added that it was apparent that some research scientists were completely ignorant about the sexual habits of homosexuals.[14]

Coordination as a factor in effective emergency research became an increasingly compelling argument as scientific information about AIDS grew. Six years into the epidemic, the president's budget announced a "major policy initiative" to coordinate federal AIDS activities:

An AIDS coordinator will improve research flexibility and the coordination of the multifaceted AIDS program. HHS's AIDS spending plans could be adjusted more easily in response to emerging research and control opportunities. Establishment of an AIDS coordination office is consistent with congressional appeals for an AIDS "czar."[15]

The federal government finally assumed an active role in the management and funding of AIDS efforts by its decision to channel all AIDS funds through an office of HHS and to appoint a full-time coordinator in the office of the assistant secretary of health. As one of six national major policy initiatives in the FY87 budget, AIDS had become a mainstream political issue. But not everyone was happy with this effort. Some NIH officials were concerned that the scheme would add a layer of bureaucracy in AIDS research and exacerbate interagency rivalries over funding. And the decision to rotate the AIDS coordinator appointment among representatives of different PHS agencies augured poorly for a successful coordination effort. Amusingly, the second AIDS coordinator was selected from CDC when NIH could not decide whom to appoint from their ranks and so nominated a CDC official. Nevertheless, the policy of rotation deserved to be revisited.

The early AIDS experience showed that the NIH intramural program was easier to redirect than the extramural program. Therefore, in an effective health emergency model, only intramural federal resources would be initially retargeted, while the extramural scientific community would be tapped for its knowledge and ideas. This strategy can be justified scientifically, for it draws on broad expertise, and administratively, because researchers who are federal employees have different obligations from scientists whose primary responsibilities are to research and teaching institutions. Plans to finance new extramural activities as the emergency continues, however, should remain on the agenda.

The OTA report on research and public health policy delineated institutional barriers that prevented the PHS from effectively mounting an attack on AIDS by using both research and health care services. The problem, in brief, was that health care payment and delivery belonged under HCFA and were bureau-cratically disjointed from health surveillance and research, which was a PHS responsibility.

The OTA researchers also pointed out another difficulty: the variation in costs among anti-AIDS efforts. That fact was not easy to accept. For example, some West Coast scientists com-plained (with incredulity) that $80,000 to support completely a viral reference laboratory for one year was not forthcoming, although a single epidemiological study might be budgeted for $250,000 at the same time. The data displayed in the OTA report brought home the message that not all projects cost the same, and that comparison of costs across program lines is naive and dangerous. Studies that involve people—clinical trials and epidemiologic surveys—are labor-intensive and ex-pensive. By the fall of 1985 several studies had examined the kinds of educational and social services provided at the local level and determined who footed the bills. Each of the studies showed that most of the funding came from local sources.

Coping with the Blood Banks' Problems

Another instance of the lack of overall direction in the AIDS emergency is acutely illustrated by the role the federal govern-ment played concerning public education and guidelines to protect the nation's blood supply in 1983.

Even before the viral cause of AIDS was known, it was urgent to screen blood donors who were at risk of contracting or having the disease and possibly spreading it through blood donation. Despite the low numbers of transfusion-related AIDS (estimated in the summer of 1983 as perhaps 1 in a million, as compared with 1 in 500,000 who received the wrong unit of blood), many were concerned about the spread of AIDS through transfusions.

At the August 1983 congressional hearings held by Weiss, Joseph Bove, representing the American Association of Blood Banks, registered the preoccupation of his industry. Asked what was needed to quell the public fear, Bove replied: "Information, sir, information . . . we need an ongoing and open line of information from the CDC."[16]

Bove expressed the frustration of the blood-banking community, as well as the apprehension of the general public. But he did not comment on the evident irony of the CDC's changing the free distribution of the *MMWR*—its main information channel—to subscription sales, in order to comply with budget cuts. This change took place in October 1982. In the FY84 budget about to be finalized, less than 4 percent of the AIDS budget at the PHS was designated for "educational programs."

Eighteen months later, when a kit to detect antibodies to the AIDS virus was about to be distributed, the federal government still failed to provide enough information about it and about its own role in the use of the test at the local level. The antibody test was designed to screen units of blood for possible contamination and was meant for use only in blood banks. The test was neither designed for, nor capable of being used as a diagnostic test for predicting AIDS. (In its initial early 1985 form, the test was questioned by some as even being adequate to monitor blood bank supplies.) Because of poor public education, much confusion persisted. At a meeting of PHS representatives, gay leaders, and blood bankers in late 1984, some people became convinced that persons at risk for developing AIDS would go to blood banks for antibody testing. Thus the very people whom the blood officials asked to stay away might flock to the banks in their anxiety to learn if they have been exposed. The test was not designed for this and neither were the blood banks, which feared a higher possibility of contamination. Participants at the meeting raised the idea of alternative testing sites where people could be tested under conditions that assured confidentiality and would receive information and counseling. Since the testing at the blood bank would be free (for blood donation is voluntary), the intent was that the alternative sites would also provide testing at no cost.

The proposal created an immediate problem concerning the financing and organization of the alternative sites. HHS announced an intention to provide limited seed funds for the first ninety days of a municipality's alternative test program. One commentator, Brett Cassens, representing the American Association of Physicians for Human Rights, interpreted this decision as evidence of PHS's philosophical commitment to a technical/medical solution to AIDS rather than to a health education and risk reduction program; at the same time, he saw this federal response as a rapid and decisive move.[17] Others saw it as a Band-Aid solution to an escalating issue that might well have been avoided by a proactive and early public campaign explaining why a blood test was being developed and what the results would mean. In matters of technology transfer, public education, and payment for implementation and counseling, policy development followed rather than anticipated the needs.

Gaps in Planning

The problems of financing research for AIDS therapies and paying for patient health services merged in the clinical attempts to treat AIDS patients during the first half of the 1980s. This merger—a hallmark of the first period of a novel health emergency—raised several issues that still awaited comprehensive policy development as the epidemic moved into its sixth year. First was the need to elaborate guidelines for Medicaid payments of costs associated with experimental therapies. Also needed were more effective mechanisms for organizing clinical trials. In addition, it was urgent to determine a policy for treating patients with AIDS Related Complex (ARC), who showed clinical manifestation of disease but did not yet have the severe constellation of symptoms that characterize the full-blown AIDS. Despite CDC estimates that there were ten times more ARC than AIDS patients, that as many as 30 to 50 percent of ARC patients might eventually develop AIDS, and that ARC patients were probably the most promising candidates for medical intervention, as 1985 ended there was neither a clear case definition of ARC for surveillance purposes, nor policy for financing ARC-related treatment.

In 1983 a diagnosis of AIDS had become accepted by the Health Care Finance Administration (HCFA) as a qualification for supplemental income, which in turn allowed eligibility for Medicaid. Medicaid payment regulations varied at the state level, however, and often did not cover experimental therapies. Analysts at HCFA attempted to estimate the fiscal impact of AIDS on federal and state Medicaid programs. Based on preliminary information gathered through the end of October 1985, federal Medicaid costs for FY86 alone were estimated at $100 million.[18] The cost to state Medicaid programs was estimated at an additional $100 million. Perhaps the most sobering aspect of these estimates was what they did not include: the costs to states and localities for payments beyond Medicaid reimbursement levels, and costs for patients who did not qualify for Medicaid; costs associated with services for ARC patients; costs of new experimental therapies, AIDS research, and supportive social services.

Similarly, although the media seemed to report, almost daily, scientific findings that might eventually lead to new drugs or vaccines, little attention was paid to the problems that were likely to face the federal establishment and the pharmaceutical industry when such biologicals were developed. In the wake of the confusion attending AIDS virus antibody testing, the need for policy planning to monitor the development of new technologies and their manufacture, licensing, and indemnification was acute.

Although the initial period of the AIDS experience provided a working model for policy development in managing a novel health emergency, the demands of the immediate crisis continued to divert attention from the set of problems that lay just around the corner, as well as from the problems that would surely accompany the next epidemic.

7

Who Is In Charge?

A LITANY of questions is often heard during a public health crisis. Are enough dollars being spent? Are the right scientists asking the correct questions? Is there an adequate research plan? What constitutes an appropriate long-range plan for research? What about coordination? How does laboratory research relate to clinical research and how are results translated into patient care? What constitutes oversight of the emergency effort? Is a congressional oversight hearing an appropriate or desirable forum for resolving these questions in the context of a real health emergency?

In each case resolution requires consensus on two levels: issues of science and issues of social policy. As the mounting volumes of congressional testimony on AIDS were clearly to show, congressional chambers with their theatrical nature were an inappropriate place to conduct a technical debate. On the other hand, an issue that *was* perfectly suited to congressional debate as a forum for mobilizing public opinion, and that required resolution before any specific question of either technical or social concern could be addressed, was the question of who should be in charge and what constitutes appropriate oversight of a health emergency effort.

Each congressional committee—whether in the House or in the Senate—has various subcommittees. An oversight subcommittee has no "line function" authority and cannot propose legislation, although it may recommend that legislation be proposed by the parent House or Senate committee. Similarly, the oversight subcommittee cannot impose sanctions. Its influence resides in its subpoena power, which allows it to delve into public and private activities in the political theatrical known as the congressional oversight hearing. The aim of the hundreds of oversight hearings held each year is either to recommend legislation or to adjust current programs by examining budgets and making budgetary recommendations.

Although congressional hearings appear spontaneous, they are carefully orchestrated events. A committee will often select witnesses whose testimony is expected to contradict that of administration officials. A draft of the administration's testimony is frequently circulated beforehand among the relevant offices of the executive branch (including OMB) for comment and to ensure consistency during the hearing.[1]

Newcomers to Washington are often confused to find only one or two members of a committee present during a hearing. The number of the committee members appearing may depend on whether the subject of discussion is of interest only to a single member's limited constituency or is of general and national concern. In addition, attendance is often determined by the extent of press coverage. Television cameras are a tremendous lure. During the sporadic hearings held on AIDS between 1982 and 1984, it was not uncommon to find either Henry Waxman or Ted Weiss presiding, with no other committee members present.

The Need for a Master Plan

One day after the Weiss hearings ended in the summer of 1984, the PHS released for public scrutiny its plan for addressing AIDS. A more elaborate AIDS Operational Plan followed in September. This second document "outlines planned activities in basic science studies, epidemiology and surveillance, testing, therapy, prevention and education." Although this was not the needed master plan coordinating AIDS activities, it did reflect the change in direction from phase one to phase two of the emergency by focusing on virus-related activities.

The 1984 planning document purposely avoided a detailed proposal for epidemiologic and experimental studies on the grounds that such protocols would undoubtedly change as data poured in. The report delineated areas that the PHS had not previously been able to target, illustrating the shift from initial to second phase concerns. These included identifying the etiologic agent responsible for AIDS, developing diagnostic tests, developing animal infection models, and seeking a vaccine and treatment. A major new PHS priority was "the transfer of this technology to health departments and medical practitioners where it will be used in the identification, prevention, and treatment of the disease."[2] The report also proposed prevention, public information, and education programs. Prominently targeted was a plan to protect blood and blood products.

Although the PHS 1984 plan was beginning to home in on the problem areas, it did not go far enough. Notably lacking was any indication of how the results of those programs were to be communicated to, funded, and used by state and local health agencies, and what effects any resultant new technology might have on the individual patient. The lack of attention to the "psychosocial implications" of the AIDS experience was to have continuing repercussions throughout 1985 and 1986 as the test to detect antibodies to the AIDS virus began to be distributed for uses the test had never been designed to address.[3]

But perhaps the report was most interesting in its admission of the need for a new approach to coordinate federal AIDS activities. Although Edward Brandt had established an internal PHS executive committee, the discovery of the AIDS virus highlighted the need for centralized control of federal programs.[4] When Brandt assumed chairmanship of a newly reorganized AIDS Executive Task Force in May 1984, a great deal of friction hampered relations between NIH and CDC and between the NCI and NIAID within NIH, in the face of mounting criticism from the extramural scientific establishment and affected communities.

Questions of Scientific Oversight

Closely allied to the question "how much research funding is enough?" is the question "how should the funds be spent?" This is another version of the perennial debate concerning oversight of the national biomedical research agenda. At one extreme is the view that only fellow scientists can judge the value of a researcher's work and determine how much and where support should be given. At the other extreme is the argument that those who provide the funds (Congress) should have a say in the amount and content of the research to be performed. Partisans of peer oversight resist the "micromanagement" of research by Congress. In contrast, legislators on Capitol Hill see oversight as a means to force accountability on the federally funded research establishment.[5] Tim Westmoreland, on Henry Waxman's staff, expressed a congressional view of NIH: "In Bethesda, they answer only to themselves and God."[6]

Four and one-half years into the epidemic, the issue of scientific oversight of the government's AIDS programs came up at a prominent scientific forum—the 1985 annual meeting of the Institute of Medicine (IOM). (The IOM is one of three national academies associated with the National Research Council.)[7] A quasi-independent, quasi-official government body, the IOM is chartered by the Congress, its members are elected by their peers from all areas related to medicine and public health, and it organizes study groups to address important issues of health policy. Like the National Academy of Sciences and the National Academy of Engineering, the institute is one of the few bodies to whom an executive branch agency can easily turn to commission a study. Such sole-source reports are generally thought to be divorced from considerations of conflict of interest, because of the unique ability of the IOM to assemble an interdisciplinary group of acknowledged experts to address problems in an apolitical way. Yet the IOM is not apolitical, in part because most IOM studies are supported with solicited funds.[8] To be sure, the conclusions of a study may not be bought in advance, and IOM retains the ability to draw its own conclusions, yet the source of funding may be an influencing factor. At any rate, the IOM's October 1985 discussion of AIDS was as interesting and political a statement as its silence had been during the initial period of the AIDS epidemic.

The annual IOM meeting is a two-day affair. The first day is reserved for a scientific symposium, and the second day for workshops where initiatives for the coming year's work are often discussed. The symposium held on October 16, 1985, in honor of IOM's outgoing president, Frederick Robbins, was entitled "AIDS: The Unfinished Story of a Virus." AIDS was the subject, in part because Robbins was a Nobel-prize-winning polio virologist and there were many parallels between AIDS and polio, and second, because AIDS was the nation's number one health priority.

The meeting also seemed to serve as a forum for a public debate on whether the PHS, and especially NIH with its mandate for fundamental research, were marshaling the full extent of the nation's scientific talent in the AIDS effort. Some members of the extramural scientific community were expressing concern that a parochial attitude at NIH—one seemingly unchecked by PHS—was beginning to affect the quality and the speed at which research progress was being made.[9] They felt that NIH decision makers were viewing the AIDS research problem as theirs alone—as a problem that would be solved solely by NIH scientists. A cynical opinion of this was that it reflected the personal ambitions of some NIH scientists to retain a predominant, perhaps exclusive, presence in the field. Such an assumption could be taken seriously only if the NIH were limiting support of extramural AIDS research by means of resource allocation and information exchange policies, while at the same time generously supporting intramural AIDS work. An "anti-extramural" policy of this sort could not be documented.

An equally chilling interpretation of the perceived parochialism was that the NIH needed to bolster its reputation in pursuit of future favorable congressional treatment. If the NIH succeeded in cracking AIDS by itself, its prestige would soar and Congress would continue to fund the institution as generously and with the limited oversight it had used in the 1960s, at the peak of its reputation as a leading research center. What happened in the following decade was the advent of genetic engineering and its commercial promise, allowing first-class scientists to command generous salaries and "perks" in academia and industry. Some of its superstars left NIH, raising fears that the institute no longer could compete for or retain the world-class researchers because of a cap on pay for federal employees. This is turn led to expressions of skepticism about whether the NIH had the effective critical mass or means of tapping America's best scientists.

The call for recruiting the best and brightest to the AIDS effort persisted. In 1985 the focus was on adequate scientific oversight of selecting and testing drugs for their potential effectiveness against AIDS. In this spirit, the organizers of the IOM's meeting may have wanted to sensitize (perhaps to jolt) the IOM membership into recognizing the urgency of AIDS, and to have them offer up collective counsel in the form of a blue-ribbon scientific oversight committee. If that was so, the plan worked perfectly: at a workshop held the second day of the annual meeting, the concept was enthusiastically endorsed. With political foresight, the IOM elected to raise the money for its AIDS study from nongovernment sources.

Before 1985 the IOM had not formally and publicly involved itself with AIDS. One reason may be that the leaders or members of the institute did not give AIDS an early high priority. Alternatively, the silence of IOM during the initial period of the epidemic may reflect a political conclusion of the institute that a low profile would complement the PHS's style and best serve the national effort. Near the end of 1982 Robbins had asked Brandt if an IOM science advisory committee could help the AIDS effort. Brandt, arguing that a single committee could not cover the "scientific waterfront" of AIDS and that IOM members were already active in PHS committees, persuaded Robbins that such an effort would not be useful.[10]

The 1985 meeting marked a significant shift toward a more active role for the IOM. In part this attitude may have reflected the perceived loss of leadership in the federal AIDS effort with the departure of Brandt from PHS, and the more general lack of leadership at HHS, where virtually all senior positions had been vacant for close to a year by the fall of 1985. In part the change at IOM may have paralleled a change in leadership at the institute itself, with the appointment of Samuel Thier as president in early 1986. Although it was two years later, the IOM appeared to respond to the 1983 majority report of the Government Operations Committee.[11] That report had concluded:

The committee believes that PHS researchers and physicians are eminently qualified to plan and conduct the nation's response to health emergencies including AIDS. At the same time, these scientists are subjected to severe political and fiscal restraints especially in times of shrinking federal budgets for public health programs . . . [Therefore] the committee recommends that an independent panel of appropriate professionals be convened to facilitate the coordination and farsighted planning of our national response to AIDS.

The debate concerning oversight of the AIDS research agenda reflects the difficulty for those in the PHS and extramural community with the requirements of phases one and two of emergency research management. In phase one, management questions center on reallocation and do not lend themselves to the leisurely processes of disciplinary peer review and consensus development normally employed in setting national research priorities. If those mechanisms are attempted, the result appears to be foot-dragging and will be criticized. In phase two questions shift to long-term planning and resource gathering for increased experimentation. These goals are more amenable to traditional decision making in the biomedical sciences.

At a seminar he chaired in January 1985 whose purpose was to "educate" the press about AIDS, David Baltimore, a Nobel Laureate in medicine, commented that the problem with AIDS research was that it was being conducted under constant public scrutiny. The frustration implicit in this remark is one more illustration of how traditional procedures are not effective during a crisis. And the fact that the IOM blue-ribbon panel was established reemphasized that the broad issues—of peer review, of how to best motivate scientists, and of how best to allocate funds to intramural and extramural programs during an emergency—remained unresolved.

The Broader Oversight Picture

Throughout the initial period of the epidemic, AIDS was defined almost exclusively as a biomedical research problem. Thus little attention was paid to the impact that the epidemic would have on the health care delivery system with regard to planning for both the provision and payment of services. Similarly unanticipated was the wave of near hysteria that swept through regions of the nation by the end of 1985. And although the central role of research was properly stressed, there was little discussion of the relation between the crisis research effort and the organization of the biomedical research enterprise during noncrisis times. This limited view—which reflected traditional institutional assignment of responsibilities—was held not only by the PHS, but also by critics in the Congress, in the press, and in the affected communities.

The OTA's "Review of the Public Health Service's Response to AIDS," released in February 1985, was a clear example of the prevailing narrow "research" perspective on the epidemic. Formally, OTA conducts studies following requests from a bipartisan group of Senate and House members. In practice, the bipartisan request is generally made after the OTA's board has been lobbied by one or several members of Congress who feel strongly that an issue needs examination. With AIDS, Ted Weiss's and Henry Waxman's staffs pushed for the study. Not surprisingly, the starting premise was that the federal effort was insufficient. And just as the administration had essentially defined AIDS as a research problem for the PHS, the subcommittee hearings and the commissioned OTA report concentrated on the organization and funding of research at NIH and

CDC. Only secondarily and in a perfunctory way did the OTA study touch upon the social implications of AIDS and the problems of organizing the federal machinery for a coordinated national effort.

As cases of AIDS increased and the cost of health service delivery began to strain local resources, debate shifted to ways to finance health services. In a manner parallel to earlier discussions of research efforts, the lack of definition of responsibility clouded the issue.

8

The Flow of Information Within the Health Establishment

CLEAR, candid, coordinated, and rapid dissemination of new findings is vital, especially during the initial stage of an emergency. Because at this stage work is a back-and-forth process, with each decision shaped by the latest findings in the laboratory, the results of public health surveillance and monitoring, and observations made by primary care providers, information must be accurate and timely. Without that, the emergency effort is slowed, even side-tracked. Yet the traditional ways of assuring accuracy are at odds with the time pressures of the health crisis.

Within the health establishment, which is composed of technical experts and generalist policy makers, communication is complicated by several factors. One of them is the time required by the traditional rules governing the presentation of new scientific information, including the slow pace of peer review and publication of technical journals. Normally, a scientist who wishes to report his findings prepares a manuscript that details the methods used, the results of the experiments, and an interpretation of the findings. When the manuscript is submitted to a journal for publication, the editor solicits critiques from several other scientists in the field to assess the accuracy and relevance of the work. The paper may then require revision and another review before publication. The review process is conducted anonymously and voluntarily, and the time elapsed from initial submission to publication can be more than year.

To eliminate this block in the flow of information, Edward Brandt requested that leading medical and scientific journals expedite the review and publication of articles concerning AIDS. Journals such as *Science, The Journal of the American Medical Association (JAMA)*, and the *New England Journal of Medicine (NEJM)* complied.[1] At *Science*, publication was accelerated in the initial period of the AIDS epidemic by having editors phone reviewers directly and assume functions often delegated to support staff. This costly and labor-intensive process was ill suited for large numbers of manuscripts. During the second period of the epidemic, as the establishment's perception of AIDS changed from an acute to a long-term disease and a chronic public health problem, the pressure for rapid publication began to lessen; in early 1986 *Science* returned to its normal publication process for AIDS-related manuscripts.

Cooperation and Competition Among Scientists

The first step in the initial period of a novel health emergency is to define the medical syndrome and to identify signs of the disease. This requires the study of blood, urine, and tissue samples obtained from patients. In the early stages of a new emergency such samples may be limited. The sharing of reagents in such short supply requires careful control, and early in the AIDS epidemic that meant deciding who would be allowed to work directly with those materials. Dr. Samuel Broder of the National Cancer Institute recalled that the shortage of specimens from AIDS patients forced the institute to "give [NCI's Robert] Gallo absolute priority over samples from the cancer institute."[2]

After the HTLV-III virus had been isolated, scientists who wanted to work with the virus requested materials from Gallo's laboratory. A number of these scientists believed that the NCI group was being less than forthcoming in the sharing of their reagents and data.[3] Even virologists at the National Institute of Allergy and Infectious Diseases were taken aback by the forms they were asked to sign before they could obtain HTLV-III samples from the NCI. Although such procedures had not previously been commonplace among medical researchers, in the early 1980s they had become so. These forms, which described the purposes and conditions for using the materials, were often essential to protect commercial and intellectual property rights. They were also used to assure that the researcher who requested the materials was fully aware of any danger associated with them. While some skeptics saw the forms as a stalling tactic, Gallo's supporters argued that the caveats were imposed for reasons of safety. After all, the AIDS virus could be lethal. Some scientists elected to try to make their own virus isolations directly from AIDS patients. The negative consequence of such attempts was that results could not be standardized because different virus isolates were being used in different labs. On the plus side, labs were forced to isolate new viruses independently, thereby providing independent confirmation of the role of human immunodeficiency viruses in AIDS and quickly finding significant diversity in aspects of the virus when isolated from different persons.

The extramural scientific community had been expressing concerns about the lack of scientific cooperation for some time. At a 1983 meeting at New York University, a spokesman from Gallo's laboratory had alluded to but refused to provide specifics about work linking a virus with AIDS. The audience reportedly booed the scientist when he refused to answer questions.[4] Yet is it not in the scientific tradition to state a conclusion without providing the evidence for scrutiny by one's peers. And because competition among scientists to be the first to find an answer is so intense, it is not unusual for a scientist not to share data until all the pieces of a puzzle have been put together. But the lethal nature of AIDS seemed to many scientists to override the usual competitive urge in favor of cooperation. The discord finally became too much to be tolerated by Public Health Service leadership. In May 1984 Brandt personally assumed the chairmanship of the PHS AIDS Executive Task Force, in part to force greater cooperation between NIH and CDC in the exchange of reagents and technical data.

In a December 1984 interview Frederick Robbins, then president of the Institute of Medicine, reflected on the parallels between the competition to find the agent that caused AIDS—particularly among scientists at NIH and CDC—and the fierce interpersonal rivalries between Albert Sabin and Jonas Salk during the development of polio vaccine:

One of the problems that is obvious now is the difficulty in coordinating the effort within our government. I know he has been criticized, but in his quiet way, I think Ed [Brandt] has done a pretty good job. Nobody can coordinate perfectly when you are dealing with ambitious young people and I suppose Gallo is in the mold of Sabin and Salk . . . anxious to make their mark. [Furthermore,] The CDC and the NIH coordination has obviously had great difficulties. The CDC found it easier to work with the French than they did with the NIH. Well, I know for a fact that Ed Brandt has beaten their heads together. He hasn't been, well, he's been somewhat effective.[5]

Frederick Robbins, who shared a Nobel Prize in 1954 with Thomas H. Weller and John F. Enders for work directly relevant to the conquest of polio, was eminently qualified to see the parallels in research between these two diseases. The work that earned the three scientists their award allowed for the growth of large quantities of polio virus in the lab, thus facilitating the development of a polio vaccine. The polio experience also established a precedent for awarding a Nobel Prize for technical advances that seemed similar to one of the problems in AIDS research (that is, growing virus in quantity in the lab). This precedent, and the lure of the Nobel Prize in contemporary biomedical circles—often called "Nobelitis"—has been interpreted as a perverse incentive underlying extreme competition in AIDS research.

There was no clear policy—and certainly no means of enforcement—for sharing results and materials among researchers; in fact, the common approach to scientific enterprise provided disincentives to the early sharing of information. The problem for research managers was to promote cooperation and rapid information exchange without stifling the competition.

The AIDS Antibody Test Kits

All drug, biological, and medical products to be marketed in the United States must first be approved by the FDA. The review process, which includes study of production details as well as product testing, is lengthy and confidential. The FDA is forbidden by law from disclosing details of the manufacturing process. This procedure thus balances the government's "need to know" with industry's need to maintain trade secrets, and it works effectively in noncrisis times. During a novel health emergency, however, the regulatory process, with its long assessment and built-in respect for industry's needs, may itself become an impediment to the research effort. The conflict between crisis management and normal "business-as-usual" patterns is illustrated by the following account of a government-sponsored workshop to assess the ELISA (enzyme-linked immunosorbent assay) test kits developed to detect antibodies to the AIDS virus in blood.

Immediately following the acceptance of a virus as a causative agent of AIDS, the PHS began planning for a simple laboratory test to detect carriers of the viral agent. Although the idea for the test was not novel—ELISAs had become standard tests during the preceding ten years and were used in various circumstances—the latest test was unique in its specificity for detecting antibody to the AIDS virus. The federal government was awarded a patent for the test in May 1985.[6] The HHS licensed five companies to develop and mass produce ELISA kits. By summer 1985 several of the federally underwritten tests were in use, and several firms that had not received a government license had developed tests of their own.

In July the FDA, CDC, and NIH jointly sponsored a workshop entitled "Experience with HTLV-III Antibody Testing—Update on Screening: Laboratory and Epidemiologic Correlations" to assess the comparative effectiveness of the different commercial test kits as well as the results obtained. The morning session was a standard scientific meeting; experiences in the blood banking and research communities were described in detail.

The afternoon session was to include presentations by manufacturers of HTLV-III Antibody test kits.[7]

It was known that the results obtained by using the various kits were not the same. The urgent questions were about test reliability, and whether the rates of false positive and false negative findings were comparable among commercial kits. In AIDS it was especially vital to establish confidence in test results, for in the absence of medical treatment for the fatal disease, the knowledge of a positive antibody test was certain to be profoundly disquieting to the patient. The test manufacturers' presentations were thus expected to provide guidance on which tests should be employed, and what kind of confirmatory tests or technical improvements were needed. Reassuringly, each presentation began with a corporate pledge to serve the American public, mankind, and science. Generalizations followed ("ours is a very reliable test with great sensitivity and specificity"). But nothing was said in public to promote legitimate scientific assessment of the tests. The problem was not one of deliberate obfuscation but of unwillingness to present confidential business information. The details that would allow for careful technical comparison of the various tests would also reveal manufacturing processes, whereas confidentiality was the key to maintaining a competitive position.

Clearly, there was a call for guidelines that could balance the protection of legitimate trade secrets and the special information requirements of the health emergency. The fact that these manufacturing processes were in part developed with public funds through limited licensing agreements further complicated the equation. Yet no precedent could be found for such guidelines, nor a context in which they might logically be developed, nor leadership to spark the effort.

Liaison with the Groups at Risk

During an evolving health emergency information changes constantly and the experts may not be able to reach consensus, so the policy maker does not know whom to listen to. In addition, he must decide how much information is enough to formulate a new policy. Some generalist policy makers, like the assistant secretary for health, will bring to their jobs a professional background in health. But even the best trained can claim expertise in only a few areas. The same problems of how much information is enough and who can be trusted occur when information is exchanged between the health research establishment and other government policy makers, such as congressmen, governors, and mayors.

Ideally, the decision of what policy to follow is based on weighing all information and all options for action. But two questions arise. Whose advice should be taken when opinions differ, especially when information is continually evolving? Can one be certain that the information represents all perspectives on the emergency? Early in the AIDS crisis one valuable asset— the views of the affected communities and much relevant information they could have offered (how best to collect data in the homosexual community; effective ways to spread health education; how best to identify negative social consequences of new policies)—was neglected by the health establishment.

In assessing his leadership of the AIDS effort, Brandt concluded that he should have opened channels of communication with the homosexual community earlier. The failure to do so was not the result of a decision to exclude this group, but rather inattention to the possibility that the group had a distinct perspective that might help the effort. In AIDS, consultation with the early at-risk groups was especially important because they were not in the social mainstream. The health officials had little understanding of the behavioral patterns and social habits that encouraged the spread of the disease, so they were unable to determine what preventive measures might be effective. Thus risk groups themselves may represent sources of information needed by health emergency managers.

The failure to consult the affected group is not unique to the AIDS experience. It is characteristic of paternalistic traditions in medicine. Physicians have not been trained to consult their patients for advice in the management of the patient's disease.

Only in recent years has a movement developed in American health care that encourages the patient to be an informed consumer. In a similar sense, as health comes to be seen more as an individual's responsibility—for example, in personal decisions over diet, smoking, and behavior—the relations between the physician and the patient and the establishment and the risk group change.

Despite the good move to include patients in the strategic planning of a health defense, political or ideological concerns may hamper consultation of affected groups. A reactionary debate ensued in the summer of 1987 concerning the appointment of a homosexual to a presidential commission on AIDS.[8] Hardline right-wingers on the White House domestic policy staff asserted that no representative of the gay community would be appointed. Although one of the twelve commissioners chosen was an avowed homosexual, the debate illustrated that even lessons already taught in the course of the same health crisis often need to be learned again.

9

Communicating with the Public

GOVERNMENT officials, professional health associations, and the media all commissioned polls to determine what the public knew about AIDS. A Roper poll taken as early as August 1983 reported that nine out of ten adults claimed to be aware of AIDS. Yet in September 1985, 52 percent of those polled by the *Washington Post*/ABC News said they knew little or nothing about AIDS. As late as January 1986, a poll released by the American Association of Blood Banks showed that 34 percent of those polled considered it likely that someone could get AIDS from a blood donation! This strange notion was widely held even though nobody had ever contracted AIDS by donating blood, and it persisted after the risk of contracting AIDS by receiving a transfusion was virtually eliminated once HTLV-III antibody screening began in American blood banks in the summer of 1985.

The polls showed that the public's understanding of AIDS was poor and its fear great. The Institute for Health Policy Analysis noted in a study released in October 1985:

Presenting poll data, which is difficult to interpret and may be distorted because of various internal biases, is one of many challenges journalists face in reporting on AIDS and other health risks. Another is for reporters and editors to be alert enough to recognize that health risks such as AIDS are newsworthy before they befall someone like Rock Hudson. Once the story is catapulted onto page one, the problem quickly becomes one of overcoverage rather than undercoverage, which, irrespective of the quality of the reporting, can contribute to an atmosphere of exaggerated concern if not panic and demands increased attention to quality of reporting.[1]

Public misperceptions about AIDS underline communication problems in the complex, vast, and highly competitive public information system known as the media. Rational explanation of the origin of public misinformation can be derived from assessing the answers to several central questions: Who speaks for the health establishment? Who listens and interprets for the media? What are the conflicts between the traditions of a free press and the caution of those managing the health emergency? How does the presentation of the news affect the management of a health emergency?

AIDS in the Media

The public learns about events in the biomedical research establishment through radio and television, daily newspapers, and weekly magazines such as *Time* and *Newsweek*. In recent years popular science magazines have provided an additional source of information. Nevertheless, the nightly news and the morning paper are still the most common sources.

Following the April 1985 International Conference on AIDS in Atlanta a veteran medical journalist was reported to say that it was like going to an orgy and not knowing where to start, or perhaps a better analogy would be going to an orgy and finding oneself impotent.[2] Reporters had more problems than just choosing which of many research results to select for their stories. They also had to decide how to report on the social context in which AIDS was being discussed: the accusations and counteraccusations by and against the groups at risk. For example, the opening sessions of the Atlanta conference came under fire from the gay community, breaking a story of deep suspicion concerning the efforts of the federal government to address a disease that predominantly affected persons who were often socially stigmatized.

The conference in Atlanta was kicked off with HHS Secretary

Margaret Heckler's keynote address. Despite its upbeat tone, Heckler's speech initiated an avalanche of negative publicity for the PHS. At an impromptu press conference following the address, some homosexual and lesbian leaders criticized the administration's priorities: Heckler was heard to state that finding a cure for AIDS had become urgent and was needed before the disease could "spread from them to us!" Such a position would naturally be unacceptable to representatives of the groups who were first and most urgently at risk for developing AIDS. And undoubtedly that was the message that came across to gay and lesbian organizers of the press conference called in response to Heckler's remarks. But what the secretary really said was:

> For individuals in every country who fall within the risk categories, AIDS is an enormously serious disease. We must conquer it for their sake. We must conquer it as well before it affects the heterosexual population and threatens the health of our general population.[3]

The intense reaction to this statement reflected the low expectations each group had come to have of the other. At a minimum, this experience indicates the difficulty of communicating both research results and research policy in a charged atmosphere.

One of the interesting stories in the AIDS epidemic is the role of the press. The press has been variously accused of underplaying the story, creating public anxiety, and spreading false information. One way to assess the role of the press in public understanding of AIDS and in shaping public policy is to examine the news stories about the epidemic in selected newspapers and journals.

Coverage of any subject can be quantified by computerized catalogues (data bases) of the contents of a selected set of newspapers or magazines. But information can be recovered from a data base only by key words assigned to an article when it is catalogued. For stories about AIDS, the logical key words are "AIDS" or "acquired immune deficiency syndrome." Of necessity, this correlation limits the period and the area that can be examined because the term AIDS was not coined until the fall of 1981, and the early reports found in newspapers directed to the homosexual community and the San Francisco newspapers referred only to Kaposi's sarcoma and opportunistic infections. Omissions, however, were not a factor with the establishment East Coast press, whose early disinterest in AIDS as a news story has been the subject of criticism. For although more than 800 AIDS cases were reported by the CDC in the early summer of 1982, the first record of a news story about AIDS in the National Newspaper Index[4] appeared only in July of that year. Although a few short pieces on Kaposi's sarcoma had run on the inside pages of the *New York Times* and the *Wall Street Journal* in 1981, data base listings show that the establishment press—as measured by the National Newspaper Index— was slow to carry the news about this disease (Figure 4).

AIDS initially was seen as a local story. Early routine coverage of the disease by the San Francisco press reflected the position of the homosexual community in the mainstream of that city. On the East Coast, news about AIDS appeared only in papers with a homosexual readership. Critics in the homosexual community accused the establishment press of not wanting to report stories about a "gay disease" until the disease was reported to affect other segments of the society. During all of 1982 only nine articles were published about AIDS. Then in December of that year AIDS was linked to blood transfusions, and ten articles appeared in January and February 1983. In May the *JAMA* scientific reports on pediatric cases and Brandt's labeling of AIDS as the nation's number one health priority led to thirty-seven newspaper articles in June 1983 alone; 103 in May, June, and July. By September coverage had dropped again and only twelve articles appeared in the National Newspaper Index's five papers. Coverage clearly was episodic and related to "news events." But AIDS stories were increasingly a subject of interest, and between February 1985 and February 1986 alone press coverage was more than double that of the previous two years.

Magazines began running AIDS stories several months before the establishment newspapers (July 1982 as against November 1982).[5] The very first article appearing in the Magazine Index

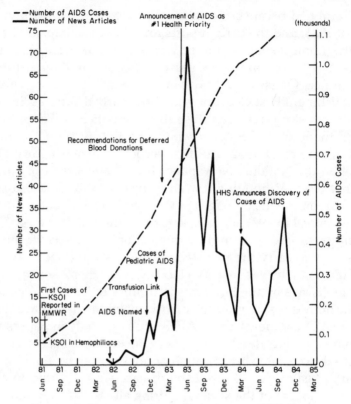

Figure 4. News Articles in Relation to AIDS Cases

was "The Gay Plague" by Michael VerMeulen, in the May 31, 1982, issue of *New York* magazine. Between summer 1982 and the end of 1984 (the mid-1983 blood scare excepted), magazines focused on personal interest and "distress" stories and on technical reviews of research, while newspapers carried a wider spectrum, with personal interest stories interspersed with policy and news events. Not surprisingly, scholarly interest in AIDS as a social phenomenon did not appear to develop until mid-1985. Also not surprising was the explosion of technical information about AIDS that fed the popular press. Judging by the contents of biomedical research journals, the mass of research reports was keeping pace with the rapid growth of cases recorded by the CDC.

One of the first writers to report the medical facts of AIDS for the layman was Lawrence Mass, a physician writing for the New York homosexual press. At the time he began covering the story, in 1981, virtually no medical-scientific articles had been written for the lay public. Between 1981 and 1983 Mass wrote over twenty stories and played a dual role of "trying to be politically active and urge active participation and politicization; and then writing to inform, report and educate."[6] His account of the commission he received from the *Village Voice* to write an article on AIDS illustrates the particular angle from which the mainstream press was willing to approach the subject of AIDS.

I was commissioned to do this piece for the *Voice*. I worked on it for about a month and it was an objective, academic, clinical, cold piece called "The Most Important New Public Health Problem in the United States" . . . a direct quote from Jim Curran, who had been calling it [AIDS] for three or four months . . .

The *Village Voice* finally rejected my piece as "not a *Voice* piece." They wanted a real human interest kind of thing that would begin by saying, "Johnny lives alone at such and such a place. There's nothing in his refrigerator but two cans of beer and a bottle of pop," or something where "fuck" is in every other sentence. I was writing this clinical news report and they didn't want that. I said, "I don't care what you do, but get this information into the paper in a major way." They waited yet another year before they published their first big feature story which was precisely that—someone has AIDS or pre-AIDS and how they are living with it. But the basic facts were still not getting out to the public.[7]

Ironically, later in the epidemic when the mainstream New York papers were covering AIDS extensively, some members of the homosexual community criticized their coverage for approaching AIDS too much as a science and medicine story and too little as a human interest and political story. For example, Dennis Altman singled out the *New York Times* for criticism in his analysis of the mainstream press's response to AIDS:

A particular grievance has long been felt against the *New York Times*, which has consistently refused to use the term "gay" and has been very remiss in its coverage of gay political and cultural events. The *Times*'s attitude seemed typified in its failure to report GMHC's [Gay Men's Health Crisis] April 1983 Madison Square Garden fund-raiser [for AIDS research], which was attended by 18,000 people, including Mayor Koch. This omission led to pickets, calls for a boycott, and a meeting between gay leaders and the vice-chairman of the newspaper.[8]

In retrospect, editors, reporters, and independent analysts attributed the early reluctance of the press to cover AIDS-related stories in part to editorial decisions about what sells newspapers: AIDS was not considered material of general interest. For example, Jerry Bishop, a veteran science reporter for the *Wall Street Journal*, ended up publishing a story in *Discover*[9] magazine on a free-lance basis when his own paper repeatedly rejected his proposal. Adding to his frustration was the time it took: *Discover* accepted the article in April 1982 and published it in September 1982—a long lead time. And to cap it all, by then the *Journal* had reconsidered its policy and published the first feature article on AIDS at about the same time.[10]

In another insight on the lack of press coverage, Lawrence Mass suggested that early resistance of the mainstream press to covering AIDS was in part due to homophobia and prejudice, whereas the initial reluctance of the homosexual press was in part denial and in part ambivalence about the implications of AIDS for sexual liberation.[11] Indeed, some of the very behavior that had been encouraged by the sexual revolution and gay liberation movements of the 1960s now had to be avoided to stem the spread of the lethal new disease.

How Science Reaches the Public

The media face a difficult task in deciding who their sources of information will be within the health research establishment. Different "experts" can provide conflicting stories. If the media report the various views with equal weight, a confusing picture may emerge.

In the early spring of 1984 a rumor circulated among the

Washington press corps that the Department of Health and Human Services had issued a "gag order" on information about AIDS. Department officials denied this and said that they were only enforcing long-established but infrequently used procedures, which called for having press interviews of scientists confirmed in writing and referring all inquiries to a central information service. The justification for a central spokesman was to enable the PHS to speak with one voice, to take the press "off the scientists' backs," and to avoid premature publication of results before they had been scientifically validated.

But usual procedures to ensure orderly flow of information seemed to be seldom employed, and even if the PHS had a policy to share technical information quickly, its officials appeared to have neither the interest nor the means of enforcing such a policy. For example, at the October 1985 IOM meetings, Robert Bazell, a reporter for NBC, asked a panel that included Robert Gallo and James Curran to comment on a manuscript of Gallo's that had not yet appeared in the *JAMA* but that had been distributed to the press in advance of publication; it examined the role of HTLV-III-infected prostitutes in the spread of AIDS.[12] The reporter wanted to know whether this report might foster public panic. Gallo said that the public response would depend on the nature of the press coverage. Curran remarked that he could not comment because he hadn't read the paper, and that the press had more access to Gallo's data than did the scientific community.

The question about the public response to the news of heterosexual transmission of AIDS was very much on target. By the spring of 1983 scientists had found cases of AIDS transmission by either homosexual or heterosexual sex, and by direct contacts with blood or blood products containing the AIDS virus. The growing—but still small—number of women raised the possibility that the proportion of men to women with AIDS might change, and questions about how easily the disease might spread from women to men and how quickly AIDS might reach a widening population.

Scientific concerns centered on identifying the risk factors that might be associated with heterosexual sex. The first studies compared prostitution (as a surrogate for having a large number of sex partners) and the frequency of sex as risk factors with earlier studies of sexual activity among homosexual men. Worry that AIDS might be readily transmitted by vaginal intercourse grew in 1983 when discrepancies emerged in the demographics of AIDS in Africa, Europe, and the United States. Among central Africans and African immigrants to Western Europe, AIDS was distributed equally among men and women. To explore the reasons for these differing demographics, PHS scientists conducted epidemiologic investigations in Zaire, using the HTLV-III antibody test.

The premature—and out of context—publicity given to the preliminary data from these studies caused widespread and unfounded alarm in the United States. A paper entitled "Household Transmission of HTLV-III in Zaire" was to be presented at the International Conference on AIDS on April 14, 1985, in Atlanta by Dr. Jonathan Mann of the CDC. On April 11 another CDC scientist, Dr. Joseph McCormick, gave a lecture at the University of California in Berkeley, during which he mentioned the preliminary results of the Zairian study. In the audience was a reporter from the *San Jose Mercury News*. The following day an article appeared in that paper claiming: "Household Transmission of AIDS Found in Africa."

The CDC study had shown only that African household members who lived with an AIDS patient were three times more likely to develop AIDS than those who did not live with an AIDS patient. In contrast, similar studies conducted in the United States showed clearly that there was no increased risk among household contacts of AIDS patients. The only logical conclusion was that some other factor was at work in Zairian households that was lacking in the United States (possibilities included sanitation, ritualistic practices such as scarification and bloodletting, a different viral agent, different sexual practices, or unknown factors, but not casual contact). The scientists reporting the work were careful not to attribute a cause to their findings. But the *San Jose Mercury News* report raised alarm by spreading an unsubstantiated message that transmission of AIDS could occur by casual contact, and deflected attention from the real risks of AIDS transmission.

Earlier in the AIDS experience similar alarmist failures in communication surrounded reports of the isolation of HTLV-III from the tears and saliva of a patient with AIDS. The public received the impression that the government's often repeated statement, "AIDS is spread by sharing bodily fluids," extended to all bodily fluids equally, including tears and saliva. Without interpretation, this extension appeared logical. Yet the preponderance of data documented months later in medical journals showed that only contaminated blood and semen were effective routes of transmission.[13]

In discussing McCormick's lecture, Donald Berreth, director of CDC's Office of Public Affairs, noted that "laboratory scientists who work with AIDS may be expert laboratorians, but that doesn't make them experts in the disease and its public health implications."[14] Berreth's comments highlight extremely difficult issues about how much the public needs to know, who should inform the public, and when the public should be told. Health professionals have different answers to these questions. When asked in December 1984 if the public knew enough about AIDS, Kenneth Sell, then scientific director of NIAID, said, "The public knows more than it needs to know about AIDS."[15] In contrast, then director of CDC James Mason said one month later: "I think there's a big gap in the knowledge. I think there are fears and concerns that are probably unfounded, and I find with every disease problem, there's as much mis-information as there is information. I'm not even sure the high-risk groups really have the information they need."[16] Although Mason recognized the need for effective public education, the PHS was not able—even when he assumed the acting directorship of the PHS in January 1985—to solve the problem, for lack of clear authority and resources.

All these examples, and many more (including the furor over the *JAMA* studies of children in households at risk; see Chapter 1), reiterate several points. First, the simplification of technical material as it goes through the media for presentation to the public can result in its complete distortion. Second, matters that appear neutral to scientists may have highly offensive connotations to one segment of the public or another, including the groups at highest risk. And third, professional medical literature is read by a wider audience than it is aimed for—a readership that may easily lose sight of important caveats like "maybe" and "possibly."

The difficulties of public presentation also stymied health officials in an area where much could be done: sex education. As the AIDS epidemic entered its fifth year, educational efforts aimed at modifying sexual behavior (thereby reducing risk of exposure to the viral agent) remained the most effective preventive health strategy. But explicit information concerning sexual transmission of AIDS was the subject of fierce contention. In July 1985 the CDC announced its intention to fund new approaches to public education in order to reduce risk. Because this goal meant changing sexual behavior, accurate and explicit information on sexuality and sexual practices—which might seem pornographic to some—was essential.

By the end of October several proposals had been reviewed and approved. Investigators had been notified informally that support would soon be forthcoming, yet several months later they were still waiting for funding. The ostensible reason was that the funds had been FY85 year-end money that no longer could be spent. But the bottleneck appeared to be created by uncertainty, debated at the cabinet level, over the kinds of information that the federal government could appropriately communicate to the public.

Besides sex, another taboo of federal public health efforts was the termination of pregnancy. In early December 1985 the CDC issued guidelines concerning the risk to the unborn fetus of a woman infected with AIDS virus, but skirted the issue of abortion by advising against pregnancy and breast-feeding. Only in 1987 did Surgeon General C. Everett Koop take a public stand with the majority of public health officials to encourage that abortion be listed as an option for a pregnant woman who was infected with the AIDS virus, as he had done a year earlier in calling for explicit sex education. Yet despite the consensus among public health officials,[17] other administration officials, most prominently Secretary of Education William Bennett, espousing conservative ideology, disputed whether such recommendations were prudent public health policy.[18]

Experts and Counterexperts

The identification by the press of the experts who speak for the scientific community plays a decisive role in communications with the public. Because individuals tend to be asked over and over again—certain names appear with regularity on the rosters of science experts testifying before Congress, for example—their interests can affect the type of information that is given out. The media star experts exert their influence within the PHS, in the Congress, and upon the press. Early in the epidemic, Anthony Fauci, then a clinical scientist at NIAID, and James Curran at the CDC were frequently consulted personally by the assistant secretary of health. Both of these civil servants also provided extensive congressional testimony. These men had responsibility for federal AIDS activities in their agencies, and their emergence as public experts on AIDS is easy to understand. It is more difficult to understand how scientists who were not as closely or officially involved in the AIDS crisis achieved superstar status and credibility among policy makers and the press.

Whom the press listens to in covering an evolving epidemic and how star status affects the reporting of scientific findings that have not been peer-reviewed are critical questions with respect to the information the public receives. The subject has been debated in the science writers' fraternity:

In the case of AIDS, the CDC's own *MMWR* [*Morbidity and Mortality Weekly Reports*] provides another quick outlet for publishing new information and disseminating it widely. Unfortunately, some scientists have been reluctant to have their findings published there, preferring instead to wait months for acceptance in a more prestigious journal . . . freedom of the press requires that each of us act independently to get the news and get it right. If we choose to report on research before it has been peer-reviewed, we should not only report the findings but also check out the principal investigator, seek the views of other scientists, and consider how it affects the public.[19]

The short memory of the press—and their readers—means that writers have little incentive to assume responsibility for accuracy or consistency. Some members of the science press have themselves called for professional restraint, however, even suggesting that the very nature of the press precludes its use as a vehicle for providing continuous, complete, and accurate information, and therefore arguing for a federal communications office to come into play. Others have suggested that stories about AIDS should be written only by people trained in medical journalism.[20]

When "expert" opinion contradicts the government's position, public skepticism and confusion result. Often only another expert can tell whether facts presented to support a position are correct. This is especially true when the speaker's credibility rests on his professional background or position (which may not be relevant to the issue). For example, not all MDs are trained in epidemiology and public health. Yet a layperson may assume that any physician's opinion is as expert as another's.

Following CDC's publication of guidelines for school-age children with AIDS,[21] the *Washington Post* ran an op-ed piece on August 8, 1985, entitled "Worry about Survival of Society First; Then AIDS Victims' Rights," which was picked up by newspapers across the country. Richard Restak, the author of the article, was identified as "a Washington neurologist who has been studying AIDS as a brain-related disease [and] is the author of *The Brain*." Restak's piece began provocatively by playing to public skepticism about the government's ability to manage AIDS: "What is new are efforts by medically unsophisticated politicians and attorneys to dictate policy in regard to an illness that has the potential for wreaking a devastation such as has not been encountered on this planet in hundreds of years." Effective measures such as quarantine were not being taken, the article continued, because of the inappropriate emphasis on the victims' rights rather than public health needs:

The AIDS victims' "rights" in these areas, we are told, should take precedence over the so far incompletely determined potential for these victims to spread this dread illness.

But what some are describing as "discrimination" and "segregation" has a long and not inglorious history in medicine. Quarantines have been very effective in beating outbreaks of scarlet fever, smallpox and typhoid in the century. Indeed, by protecting the well from the ill we follow a long-established sensible and ultimately compassionate course. Throughout history true humanitarianism has traditionally involved the compassionate but firm segregation of those afflicted with communicable disease from the well. By carrying out such a policy, diseases have been contained.

The piece conveyed the impression that the CDC's guidelines on school-age children with AIDS were misguided, based on a misunderstanding of the spread of infectious disease and promoted by ill-informed officials.

Restak's piece presents a version of "the hunt for the AIDS smoking gun" wherein government villains were attempting to protect the minority's rights at the expense of mankind's health. On the surface, Restak's argument is appealing—unless one knows the facts about the development of federal AIDS policy, has an accurate understanding of the history of quarantine, and is aware of the many routes by which infectious diseases can be transmitted.

Some of the most prestigious professional positions in public health are found in government service. It would be hard to find a greater repository of information on the spread of infectious disease or a wider understanding of the difficulties of disease management than at the CDC. During the first years of the AIDS epidemic, it was the explicit strategy of the PHS to leave AIDS policy formulation to the medical experts.

Therefore attribution of AIDS policy formulation to "medical ignoranti" rings false.

Moreover, by the time the guidelines for children with AIDS in school were published in 1985, it was well known that AIDS was not spread by casual contact—a fact documented by antibody screening of household contacts of AIDS patients and health care workers taking care of AIDS patients. However, the antibody screening data on which CDC based its arguments had not yet appeared in the professional literature nor in the *MMWR*. The scientific community was being asked to accept conclusions without having direct access to the supporting data. Thus the skepticism about the government's ability to make the right decisions came in part from the absence of data available for public scrutiny.

A theme in the Restak op-ed piece was unwillingness to accept *de minimus* (negligible) risk in the case of AIDS— especially in policy concerning children. The concepts of *de minimus* and comparative risk are difficult to convey to the public. Thus in response to public outcry—in part attending Restak's piece—James Mason, then acting assistant secretary for health, stated: "The risk to a child from a schoolmate with AIDS was far less than the possibility of the child sustaining an accident on a school bus when the bus was hit by lightning."[22] Science could not, however, provide an absolute guarantee that there could be "no" risk associated with children with AIDS or that it was totally impossible for a mosquito to transmit the disease. The scientific method requires first the formulation of an hypothesis; experiments are then designed to test the validity of the hypothesis. An experiment could not be designed to guarantee that an unlikely event would never occur. The best that could be done experimentally was to look for positive evidence of disease transmission. But arguments based on negative data are always susceptible to disbelief, and in the AIDS crisis they were unacceptable because the consequences of the disease were so terrifying.

As for quarantine, historically it had been employed appropriately under some circumstances and inappropriately at other times.[23] It would not be logical to use quarantine for stemming the spread of AIDS, however, because this is not a disease that is casually transmitted. Even if there were a scientifically defensible reason to consider quarantine for AIDS, to implement it would be impractical and too costly. For in August 1985 between one and two million Americans (approximately 1 in every 200) were estimated to be infected with the AIDS virus, and thus potentially able to transmit the disease to others.

Unfortunately, public opinion polls continued to express public confusion on matters of transmission. A *New York Times* poll of September 1985 said that ninety-eight percent of Americans knew that AIDS was a critical health problem. Forty-seven percent said they knew that the disease was easily and casually transmitted. The message that AIDS is difficult to contract except by exchange of semen and blood was not getting across. An article in the *New York Times* of December 20, 1985, reported that: "A majority of Americans favor the quarantine of AIDS patients, and some would embrace measures as drastic as using tattoos to mark those with the deadly disorder, according to a poll published today."[24]

Bias and the Press

Just as the way in which the health establishment presents information affects press coverage, the bias of the press affects interpretation of events. The natural tendency is to select information that supports preconceived notions—and it is a tendency that is difficult to counter. One example on the other side of the ideological spectrum from the piece in the *Washington Post* is an article in *Harper's* magazine, which gave the opposite interpretation to the public health officials' statements that AIDS is not casually transmitted and that the best defense against the disease was for individuals to follow safe-sex guidelines.

On March 10, 1985, Lewis H. Lapham, editor of *Harper's* magazine, participated in a Sunday morning television news program produced by WPIX, in New York City. Moderated by Richard Heffner, the program included Dr. Mathilde Krim, director of the AIDS Medical Research Foundation, and Diane

Camper, of *The New York Times* editorial board. Lapham, who had previously taken only an intelligent layman's interest in AIDS, arrived for the taping with information culled from daily press items and from David Black's article in the *Rolling Stone*.[25] Yet what Lapham heard during that television program led him to write an op-ed piece that was picked up by newspapers around the country.

In "AIDS and the Political Right: Smugness, But Little Help," Lapham wrote:

AIDS so conveniently fits the political and theological specifications of the Reagan administration that a prophet of the ascended right might be pardoned for welcoming it as the long-awaited scourge of God.

On a television program, I heard a doctor say with more than a hint of comfortable righteousness in her voice, that the affliction was impervious to medical science.

"No," she said, "we know of nothing that can cure it except a change of behavior. I'm sorry, but people will just have to learn to mend their ways."

It is possible that I do the doctor an injustice, which is why I refrain from mentioning her name. I know nothing of her motives, her religion or her politics, but her pious manner reminded me of the way in which the Reagan administration has elected to deal with the outbreak of AIDS. Several government spokesmen have managed to convey the unfortunate impression that the victims of the disease deserve what they get . . . here is a secular authority preaching a sermon of sexual Armageddon, and as I listened to her foretellings of doom it occurred to me that AIDS was a disease uniquely suited to the American temperament . . .

The apologists for the Republican theory of paradise at last have been armed with indisputable proof of the evil inherent in the permissiveness of the 1960s. The fear of contagion becomes their best and final weapon for quelling the spirit of sexual rebellion. Perhaps it is true that AIDS is a modern analogue of the bubonic plague known to the Middle Ages as the Black Death.

But if this is so, and if the authorities know it to be so, they should quit preaching sermons and trade the cost of at least one MX missile for research into a deadly disease said to be even more deadly than the Russian army or Fidel Castro.[26]

The article seems to touch all the rhetorical bases: accusations of knee-jerk reaction; skepticism that the federal government was truly committed to a major program for combating AIDS; the linkage of defense with health spending; and finally, characterizing PHS's request for behavioral change as merely the expression of the prevailing political ideology. Ironically, the doctor to whom Lapham attributed right-wing spokesmanship—Mathilde Krim—has often been an outspoken critic of the federal response to AIDS. Krim's AIDS Medical Research Foundation, a forerunner to the American Foundation for AIDS Research, was in part started to support the research of extramural scientists. Lapham's article, however, seemed to subscribe to the theory of an AIDS "smoking gun." In response to extensive public reaction to this inflammatory piece, Lapham organized a *"Harper's* roundtable" on AIDS.[27]

The most disturbing element in this episode is the assignment of an ideological motive to a pragmatic public health measure. The decision to encourage groups at risk for AIDS to change their sexual behavior was a medical, not a moral, judgment. Indeed, at the same time that Lapham saw sexual Armageddon, community-based organizations serving the gay population in San Francisco were circulating educational literature, some of it stating, for example, "Prevention is all we've got—and that means halting transmission of the AIDS virus."[28]

The press at opposite ends of the political spectrum continued to weigh in. A leaflet distributed in 1983 by Communistcadre, a self-styled scientific Trotskyist group, proclaimed "AIDS is political germ warfare by the U.S government."[29] In counterpoint, under headlines that shouted "Germ Warfare Nightmare Unleashed by Our Enemies!" the British tabloid *Weekly World News* claimed in January 1986: "Britain's top expert in sexual diseases has stunned the scientific world with a shocking report that AIDS is a man-made virus developed by the Soviet Union for germ warfare."[30] This fanciful discussion over who "engineered" the AIDS virus surfaced again in early spring 1987, in Moscow, in the form of rumors that the virus was the result of American germ warfare.

10

Lessons for the Future

T HE TIMELY resolution of a novel health emergency requires closely coordinated efforts by diverse institutions. Yet given the way the system functions, normal everyday operations make an efficient and integrated response to a new disease extremely difficult. Business as usual—which includes adversarial relationships between executive and congressional branches of the federal government, rivalries among different agencies within the Department of Health and Human Services, lack of clear-cut lines of authority and accountability among officials in different levels of government, and informal relations between the public and private sector—is part of the problem. Although on a day-to-day basis such practices may foster creative tension and provide checks and balances, they come in conflict with the successful handling of a novel health emergency.

Examination of the first five years of the AIDS epidemic reveals the need to liberate the managers of a novel health emergency from routine administrative, budgetary, and bureaucratic red tape. The aim of this chapter is to extract the main lessons of the initial period and to stimulate thought about how to craft an improved strategy, in the form of a federal plan, for managing future emergencies.

The second period of the AIDS epidemic shows examples of the benefits of planning in improved policy. At a meeting held to examine how to employ AIDS virus antibody tests to prevent spread of disease at the CDC in February 1987, and at another gathering to discuss vaccine development at the NIH in March

1987, the participants explored not only the state of science, but the social, financial, and legal implications of antibody testing and vaccine development. Thus companion laboratory research, public education, and social services agendas were identified. Both these exercises in strategic planning for AIDS were heartening for their contrast with the lack of planning for deployment of the first AIDS virus antibody tests in early 1985.

Despite these welcome signs that other lessons of the AIDS experience can be used in forming new policy, the continuing 1987 confrontation between the secretary of education and the surgeon general, the idiosyncratic presidential commission established in July 1987, and a proposed congressional commission on AIDS attest to the need for more unified direction. The set of guidelines that follows is a somewhat formal way of stating the conclusions that come to mind after examining the events of the early years.

1. Responsibility and leadership for managing a novel health emergency should be centralized and assigned to a federal official.

National leadership is essential for ensuring orderly and efficient coordination of health emergency efforts; clear assignment of responsibility for leading the emergency response should therefore be made early. The federal government's centralizing the responsibility in a publicly prominent and visible office can bring stature and importance to the emergency enterprise. It can tell those engaged in the effort that their work is valued, and it can assure the public of the government's commitment to solving the problem. In addition, it can provide consistent information in an orderly fashion, and thereby gain public confidence in the government's ability to get the job accomplished.

Assignment of responsibility must be accompanied by the authority to cross turf boundaries that are strictly adhered to in ordinary times. For example, when the assistant secretary for health was charged with the leadership for the federal AIDS response in 1981, his efforts were restricted to the Public Health

Service. The result was that necessary social services that should have been forthcoming through efforts of the Health Care Finance Administration, research capabilities that should have been mobilized through efforts of the National Science Foundation's constituency, programs of the military, and activities of numerous private organizations were neither marshaled, nor informed, nor coordinated with PHS efforts.

In 1985, when Congress mandated that the office of assistant secretary for health provide "overarching" coordination of efforts to combat AIDS, the more extensive mandate was still restricted to HHS activities. This was insufficient to bring together the entire anti-AIDS effort. For example, the activities of the military—whose AIDS expenditures are estimated to equal half of HHS's in FY87—were not under HHS authority. This situation results from the historic decentralization of health responsibilities among diverse branches of public and private institutions sketched in the first section of this book. Without a formal mechanism to coordinate diverse health activities during an emergency—a mechanism that does not now exist—an efficient, integrated response to a health emergency is not possible.

The person assigned leadership responsibility should command public respect, bureaucratic attention, and the respect of other health officials. Because the secretary of HHS is rarely a health professional, the leadership—which cannot be titular—would most probably be delegated to the assistant secretary for health, or a specially appointed "emergency czar." In any case, the backing of the highest levels of government is needed. Members of the IOM committee that studied the federal response to AIDS have emphasized the importance of presidential endorsement.[1] But the responsibility must be placed with knowledgeable public health professionals.

2. Generous and centralized finances, as well as flexible budget authority dedicated to the emergency effort, are needed for research, health and social services, and public education.

The effectiveness of an emergency effort depends in large part on available financial resources. The most difficult aspect of coordinating across agency and departmental lines concerns budgetary matters, and, historically, interagency efforts without central budget authority fail because they have "no teeth." The purpose of centralizing the budget is to facilitate clear accounting, to separate emergency funding from the normal budget process, and thus to speed the provision of funds and eliminate redundancy.

Three kinds of budgetary requirements arise during a novel health emergency. In the initial period, before the nature and dimension of the emergency are well understood, resources must be reallocated. Such reallocation occurs at the discretion of individual agency directors and officials at HHS headquarters in Washington. Improving regular budget operations and allowing agency directors greater flexibility and discretion will make reallocation easier. At present flexibility is severely limited by the trend toward detailed "micromanagement" of technical programs by the Office of Management and Budget (OMB) and the Congress, and by the political imperative to decrease domestic spending.

By the time a clear emergency has been recognized, consolidation and centralization of finances is needed. It is necessary to make financial provisions for unforeseen events—for instance, to have money available for capitalization on unexpected research and treatment opportunities. That is the time when supplemental funds provided by a standing contingency fund— such as the one provided by the 1983 Health Emergency Act— would be most valuable, as would a contingency allowance for additional personnel.

As of spring 1986 the contingency fund provided by the Health Emergency Act had not been employed, in part because the conditions that would allow its use and the details of administering its resources were never well defined. But the Health Emergency Act could be used in the future for preliminary and limited emergency initiatives if the enabling legislation were modified to spell out how the funds were to be administered by central emergency leadership.

Efforts requiring extraordinary resources—such as those that followed the identification of the virus that causes AIDS—are too great to be accommodated by either a standing contingency fund or a prospective annual emergency budget. An additional mechanism should be devised to meet such needs: for example, supplemental congressional appropriations that could be rapidly awarded to the leadership office. Mechanisms used by the Federal Emergency Management Agency to provide supplemental appropriations may also serve as a model. Any mechanism proposed will of course provide accountability, an essential element for minimizing disputes and ensuring public confidence.

3. Central oversight and management of research targeted to a novel health emergency must include the best scientists drawn from the government, university, and industrial sectors.

Traditionally, basic biomedical research is not narrowly focused or closely monitored, whereas work directed toward a novel health emergency is more restricted. This is a source of friction within the fundamental research community. Another area of contention is competition for financial resources. Scientific research is always limited by the availability of trained scientists, facilities, and research funds. Although resources directed to the emergency effort will not be available for other projects, the need for emergency-related research does not eliminate the need to continue work on other health problems. During a health emergency research managers must try to minimize the disruption of ongoing health research programs.

The financial and intellectual cost of stopping ongoing research, the realization that the most effective research occurs in the context of several groups of scientists, and the resistance of scientists to the concept that basic research can be targeted, raise the question whether all scientists should have equal responsibility to respond to a health emergency. If the primary responsibility lies with the federal establishment, then scientists who are also civil servants should be the first ones to shift their research directions. Moreover, the efforts of government-affiliated scientists in federal labs can be more easily centralized and coordinated than those of scientists dispersed throughout the country. The need for a large cadre of civil-servant scientists able to respond early to a novel health emergency provides a strong argument for vigorous support of fundamental research in federal facilities during normal times. In a similar sense, extramural basic research programs must be kept strong. Early scientific successes in AIDS are directly attributable to basic research programs of the 1960s and 1970s.

Early AIDS research efforts were marked by rivalries between the NIH and the CDC, and between civil-service and university-based scientists over control of the emergency research agenda. Assigning responsibility for parts of the research effort through a central office may minimize such conflicts, especially if a well-formulated process for soliciting scientific expertise is in place. The issue is not who should be involved: everyone's expertise is needed. Just as the expertise of scientists outside the government is used to assess the funding of noncrisis extramural research, such advice must be included in guiding emergency efforts taking place within national laboratory settings.

4. Strategic planning that encompasses immediate, short-term, and long-term problems is essential to successful management of a novel health emergency.

A novel health emergency demands simultaneous—not sequential—problem solving. Because the aim of research is to develop rapidly practical medical drugs, devices, and diagnostics, crisis managers must force simultaneous consideration of the basic research program, the commercial development of research results, and the use of the commercial products—including public education. This consideration must be well under way before the research solution has been found. For example, in 1982, even before the specific infectious agent of AIDS was known, PHS scientists knew that laboratory tests would be needed to screen blood. When they began targeting research for an effective blood test, they also should have begun planning for the way the tests would be used, as well as for the way of dealing with the social consequences of the tests. Neglect of strategic planning generated public confusion and discomfort with federal management of the epidemic.

A detailed strategic plan will benefit from the counsel of an interdisciplinary team of public health professionals, as well as experts in logistics, law, mass communication, education, and other fields. Representatives of the groups at high risk in any given health emergency need to be included. With AIDS, indecision about where to do antibody testing, uncertain policy regarding military personnel with positive antibody tests, and rejection of proposals to provide sterile needles and syringes in recognition of the spread of AIDS among drug addicts show clearly how inadequate attention to social, ethical, and legal questions hampers public health policy. The AIDS experience also shows that protecting an individual's rights may come in conflict with concern for the general public health. Consequently, health crisis management planning must be broad: if it can address the dozens of problems that may be anticipated, the truly unexpected ones are less likely to disrupt the emergency effort.

Any strategic plan devised for a specific crisis must be continually reevaluated—particularly the premises upon which decisions are based and projected timetables. Thus it is important to develop criteria for an evaluation team, for specialist credentials, and for the frequency of evaluations. To assure objectivity, the evaluation team must include specialists who did not participate in setting the original schedule.

5. Public education is essential and must begin early in a health emergency.

Public polls showed that even six years after the onset of the AIDS epidemic, neither the general public nor high-risk groups had a clear understanding of AIDS or of its means of transmission. The federal health establishment must improve its delivery of candid and accurate information to the public and to the press. In turn, the press should develop standards of accountability for the information it provides during an emergency.

The government can improve its performance by scheduling

frequent briefings, taking its message directly to the public through frequent advertisements in the media, and establishing the dissemination of information as a high priority. The advice of media and advertising professionals would be helpful in designing a campaign that tailors information to various risk groups in terms that will be best understood. The need to improve standards of accountability of the press during a health emergency runs into the fundamental issue of freedom of the press. Change must come from within the profession.

Public education must be concerned simultaneously with disease prevention, treatment, and cure. Educating the public requires no new legislation or authority but rather the development of new policy and allocation of sufficient resources.

A mechanism for collating and distilling research data for public consumption is essential to dispel public confusion and suspicion. Without such a mechanism, the idiosyncratic views of prominent public figures, which often prove wrong, receive as much attention as more informed opinions. In the AIDS crisis, the general misconception that AIDS could be transmitted casually arose in the absence of a consistent and clear public presentation of the facts. A national information office devoted to the emergency and linked to the central management office would have credibility to the extent that the public has confidence in federal handling of the crisis.

Early in the AIDS crisis, the public health imperative to disseminate sexually explicit information became confused with issues of morality, puritanism, pornography, and First Amendment rights. Direct federal government dissemination of such materials may be precluded by political realities. Yet the need for public health education is not diminished. Therefore, in its emergency planning, the government should acknowledge its limitations and be prepared to delegate the responsibility for education, under contract, to community organizations.

6. A response to new health emergencies must take a long view and avoid short-term solutions that may hamper management of the next emergency.

Time and again, problems in responding to the AIDS emergency were exacerbated because a more difficult problem of a general social nature had not been resolved when it originally came up. For example, the ad hoc solution to the problem of indemnification during the swine flu vaccine program now threatens the hoped-for development of a vaccine for the AIDS virus.

In 1976 the country poised for an outbreak of influenza that some experts predicted would rival the epidemic of 1918, which affected over 0.5 percent of the American population and resulted in a death toll of more than 600,000.[2] Since the 1976 flu threatened to create a similar health emergency, the federal government mounted an unprecedented crash program to produce an influenza vaccine and to immunize the greatest possible number of Americans.

Manufacturers balked at producing a vaccine without adequate testing, reasoning that they might be held liable should an inadequately tested vaccine produce unacceptable side effects. While manufacturers were willing to assume liability provided they were allowed time for proper testing, the government considered speed more important. To set the national program in motion, Congress enacted special legislation that indemnified manufacturers of the swine flu vaccine for all awards above a given amount.[3] Millions of Americans were vaccinated, some suffered unfavorable side effects, and the government found itself footing a massive bill even a decade later. During congressional debate at the time, concern was voiced and discounted that the swine flu legislation might establish an unhealthy precedent.[4]

The question of indemnification arose again in 1985, when the nation's supply of diphtheria-pertussis-tetanus (DPT) vaccine dwindled because two of the only three concerns still manufacturing the vaccine had decided to withdraw from the market. Their decision was based on small profits and fear that damage suits (encouraged by the swine flu litigation) would further decrease their profits. Arguments for federal backing to cover liability of vaccine manufacturers arose anew, but Congress rejected any indemnification plan. A vaccine bill designed to address some of the troubling product liability questions passed Congress in 1986, without resolving all the issues, however. In view of this history it is easy to predict that pharmaceutical manufacturers will be reluctant to take the risk of producing an AIDS vaccine in the absence of further safeguards provided by government.

Another set of long-term ramifications of medical problems arose over the newly developed technology to test for antibodies to the AIDS virus for insurance underwriting purposes. The test worked, but there was no knowing how a positive AIDS virus antibody test should be interpreted, because no one could determine who among those infected would get sick. Moreover, if a person's positive antibody status were known, he or she would suffer discrimination due to general fear of AIDS, possibly lose employment, and consequently lose health insurance benefits. In response to all these concerns, some states enacted law prohibiting AIDS virus antibody tests for insurance purposes, creating a patchwork rather than a single national insurance policy.[5]

Difficult unresolved ethical concerns accompany the development of new drugs. Individuals with the disease will want to avail themselves of any possible hope for cure, even when the effectiveness of the drug treatment has not been proved. To determine what drugs are useful and which ones are useless—and perhaps harmful—controlled clinical trials are necessary. Drugs being tested in such trials are called investigational new drugs (IND).

FDA establishes the rules for clinical testing and use of INDs.[6] For years, the lengthy procedures required by FDA for new drug approval have come under public fire. Although now streamlined, the process is still time-consuming. For the victim of a lethal disease, waiting for treatment until a drug has been approved might make it too late. The patient wants to take the chance of an untested drug, however risky. One of the most widely publicized quests of victims of AIDS was Rock Hudson's trip to Paris in spring 1985, for treatment with an experimental drug (HPA-23) that was not available in the United States. Although the actor subsequently died, and HPA-23 has not been found to be effective, a public outcry ensued over the restrictions on experimental drugs.

Advocacy groups demanded that, because of the fatal nature of AIDS, experimental drugs be made available on a compassionate basis. Under existing procedures physicians can request experimental drugs under the rules governing compassionate and therapeutic INDs. Some researchers feared that widespread use of these mechanisms would compromise the goal of finding an effective drug because patients might elect a compassionate use and then not volunteer to participate in clinical studies. This issue is not specific to AIDS but occurs each time a new drug is tested for a lethal disease. Other examples of unproved drugs that captured public enthusiasm are laetrile in the 1960s and interferon in the 1970s for treatment of cancer.

The issue of new drugs is emotionally charged and complicated. There is good reason on each side, and decisions must be approached with a sensitivity both to patients and to researchers, backed by a solid understanding of FDA rules and their rationale. An effective public information program, widespread voluntary participation of an informed public, and clinical trials are crucial. The alternative is political pressure to make extraordinary exceptions to the drug laws on an ad hoc basis, which would only establish precedents that, like the swine flu vaccine indemnification program, may adversely affect efforts to develop new drugs.

A Proposal for a National Novel Health Emergency Plan

When in 1986 officials of the Institute of Medicine called for the immediate appointment of a national commission to coordinate the nation's response to AIDS, they clearly recognized and reiterated the need for an overarching strategy for the emergency. Had a national plan for a novel health emergency existed, the procedures for implementing and running such a commission would have been in place. The establishment of the AIDS Commission—an ad hoc response—does not invalidate the need for a process by which such commissions could be expeditiously accomplished. The goal of a national plan is to facilitate the management of unique problems of novel health emergencies by providing a management framework that would include an emergency-specific central office with the mandate and authority for responses, resources, and attention to educational, social, and medical questions that would arise.

The first and most difficult step is to define the criteria that initiate a management framework. Without a clear picture of the dimension of the public health problem and its consequences, an emergency program cannot be set in motion. How many and what kind of warning signals make a crisis? In developing the criteria for how a plan would be initiated one must draw on lessons and models from the past.

It is also useful to examine existing plans for managing such national emergencies as floods, industrial disasters, and limited conventional warfare. For example, the Federal Emergency Management Agency (FEMA) coordinates and undertakes actions in response to diverse emergencies such as floods, plane crashes, and volcanic eruptions. But the fact that FEMA's activities are triggered by an immediately recognizable disaster only highlights the problem of knowing when to classify a novel disease as a health emergency, for unlike the crises that FEMA manages, consciousness of a novel health emergency evolves slowly. In 1986, after more than one million Americans had been exposed to the AIDS virus and more than 10,000 had died of the disease, there was little doubt that AIDS constituted an emergency. Yet only a few years earlier the idea that AIDS deserved special attention had been strongly contested, even though the assistant secretary for health and the director of CDC knew they were dealing with a health crisis.

Elaboration of a health emergency plan would benefit from examining other future-oriented studies. For example, problems in setting priorities concerning the financial aspects of vaccine development were examined in a study by the IOM done for the NIAID.[7] The study revealed how difficult it is to calculate and compare all the considerations—monetary costs, extent of human suffering, technical feasibility—that must be taken into account when allocating limited national resources for the management of programs to combat different diseases.

Members of the diverse health research establishment will join the national plan only if they can be productive in their area of expertise and if their interests are protected. The entire management scheme must take into account various sensitivities as federal, state, and local responsibilities are defined, and the details must be molded with an appreciation of the traditional divisions of power. The groups that will participate in carrying out the emergency response should be asked to participate in drawing up the plan.

A novel health emergency management plan might be formulated in the Congress through legislation, in the executive branch through rulemaking or executive order, or in a nongovernmental forum followed by congressional or executive action. But the most attractive body to draft such a plan is an independent national commission. Such a commission might be convened by the secretary of HHS (with the president's mandate) and represent the interdisciplinary skills needed for effective crisis management of novel health emergencies. The commission would be nonpartisan, operate in public view, and be prepared to issue an independent report.

Among the planners should be representatives from the Congress and HHS, state and local officials, and health professionals representing the three parts of the health research establishment. To ensure the implementation of any framework designed by a commission, legislation would be required. The legislation should spell out budget authority and how the plan would be initiated, but, to maintain flexibility, it would leave open the details of managing each aspect of an emergency.

Developing a novel health emergency plan, defining criteria for its use, and ensuring its implementation will not be simple. Once devised, any implemented plan will change as its strengths and weaknesses are revealed. But such a plan could be a vital factor in dealing successfully with the next novel health emergency. For the next time the health establishment faces a new disease of unknown cause, treatment, and cure, the search for answers to a new set of questions will again be as agonizing as the disease itself.

How much will it cost to draw up and implement a national plan for managing novel health emergencies?

We cannot know the price of an emergency; even with AIDS, figures are deceptive and difficult to interpret. The results of one part of an emergency response will affect other efforts. For example, dollars not spent on AIDS prevention through public education will undoubtedly translate into dollars spent on patient care. Figures abound in the press that estimate the costs of AIDS in 1986 alone to be at least $10 billion. But what of the cost of productive years lost to the economy by the death of thousands of young Americans? Improving the national response to an epidemic such as AIDS by means of an emergency health plan is cheap at any price.

Appendixes
Notes
Index

The Chronology of AIDS Research

This statement from Robert Gallo and Luc Montagnier constitutes part of the agreement between the U.S. and French AIDS research groups.

This history is by no means exhaustive. It outlines the main contributions of the two central parties and of some other groups to the determination of the causative agent of AIDS (acquired immune deficiency syndrome). This is not to diminish the important contribution made in this field (either independently or in collaboration with us) by other laboratories and clinicians distributed worldwide.

Both sides wish it to be known that from the beginning there has been a spirit of scientific cooperation and a free exchange of ideas, biological materials and personnel between Dr. Gallo's and Dr. Montagnier's laboratories. The spirit has never ceased despite the legal problems and will be the basis of a renewed mutual cooperation in the future.

The parties also believe that some clarification is needed regarding their position on nomenclature. Various generic names have been given to the AIDS virus. Dr. Gallo and his collaborations named it HTLV-III in their May 1984 publications according to a recommendation made in September 1983 at the Cold Spring Harbor meeting on HTLVs by a group of ten European, Japanese and American retrovirologists. They suggested that names of human retroviruses discovered in the future related to but distinct from human T-leukaemia virus be named sequentially, numbered HTLV-III, IV, and so on.

Dr. Montagnier and his collaborations first reported in May 1983 the identification of a novel human retrovirus not closely related to HTLV-I and II and in public meetings from September 1983 and

This chronology appeared in *Nature*, 326 (2 April, 1987), pp. 435–436, and is reprinted by permission of Macmillan Magazines Ltd.

153

subsequently in publications from 1984, they named this virus LAV for lymphadenopathy-associated virus because the first patient from which it was isolated had lymphadenopathy syndrome.

The US Department of Health and Human Services officially assumed a double generic name HTLV-II/LAV in recognition of the contributions of both sides.

When the genome structure of the AIDS virus was determined in 1985, the results showed some major differences in the organization of the genetic information from HTLV-I and II. This prompted another and more formal nomenclature committee to suggest a simpler and new generic name as the virus belonged to an entirely new class of human retroviruses. Their suggestion was to use the generic term HIV—human immunodeficiency virus. They also suggested maintaining specific strain names (LAV-1$_{BRU}$, LAV-1$_{LOI}$, HTLV-III$_B$, HTLV-III$_{RF}$, ARVI . . .) in the interest of continuity and appreciation of the biological differences of the strains. Both groups agree with this recommendation.

We set out a brief chronological history of some critical published facts, in the period up to May 1985, on the discovery and demonstration of AIDS as a retroviral disease.

Retroviruses

1970–73. Following Temin's hypothesis that RNA tumour viruses replicate via a provirus DNA intermediate, Temin and Mitzutani (1970),[1] and independently Baltimore (1970)[2], discover reverse transcriptase. Later, the existence and integration of infectious proviral DNA is demonstrated by Hill and Hillova (1971)[3] and confirmed by Montagnier and Vigier (1972)[4], Svoboda and co-workers (1973)[5], and others. Spiegelman (1970)[6], Gallo (1971, 1972)[7,8], Gerwin et al. (1972)[9] and others independently develop useful sensitive specific assays for reverse transcriptase of retroviruses.

1976. Morgan, Ruscetti and Gallo (1976)[10] discover T-cell growth factor, or interleukin-2 (IL-2), necessary for long-term *in vitro* cultivation of human T cells.

1979. Barre-Sinoussi, Montagnier, Lidereau, Sisman, Wood and Chermann (1979)[11] show that antibody against alpha interferon allows significant increase in mouse retrovirus production by infected cells.

Human Retroviruses

1980–82. Gallo, Poiesz and co-workers (1980) isolate[12] and (1981) characterize[13] the first human retrovirus, called human T-cell leukaemia virus type I (HTLV-I). Hinuma *et al.* (1981)[14] identify C-type virus in a cell line isolated by Miyoshi from a patient with adult T-cell leukaemia (ATL) and detect antibodies against antigen-bearing cells in patients with ATL. Yoshida and co-workers (1982)[15] isolate and characterize adult T-cell leukaemia virus (ATLV) and demonstrate clonal integration of ATLV proviral DNA in leukaemic cells of patients. In a cooperative study, Gallo and co-workers together with Miyoshi and co-workers (1982)[16] show ATLV to be identical with HTLV-I. In collaborative studies, Catovsky, Blattner, Gallo and co-workers (1982)[17,18] show HTLV-I to be a contributing aetiological factor in T-cell leukaemia in the Caribbean region. Gallo and co-workers (1982)[19] isolate a second type of retrovirus, HTLV-II, from a cell line obtained from a patient with hairy-cell leukaemia.

AIDS

1981. Gottlieb and co-workers (1982)[20], Friedman-Kien and co-workers (1981)[21], Siegel and co-workers (1981)[22], Masur and co-workers (1981)[23] and Mildvan and co-workers (1982)[24] independently diagnose a new disease, AIDS, in groups of young homosexual men.

1982. Epidemiological evidence suggesting that AIDS is a new infectious disease is developed by the Centers for Disease Control (1982)[25].

February 1983. At the Cold Spring Harbor Workshop on AIDS, Gallo proposes that AIDS is probably caused by a retrovirus, presumably a variant of HTLV-I or II.

May 1983. Barre-Sinoussi, Chermann, Montagnier and co-workers (1983)[26] publish: (1) the isolation and identification of a non-transforming retrovirus (later called lymphadenopathy-associated virus (LAV)), different from HTLV-I and HTLV-II, in cultures of T lymphocytes derived from a patient with lymph-adenopathy syndrome; (2) the continuous passage of the virus by its transient growth in cultures of T lymphocytes of normal blood donors; (3) the identification of a major protein associated with this virus, p25, not immunologically cross-reactive with the p24 of HTLV-I; and (4) the detection by immunoprecipitation of antibodies against this protein in two patients.

Essex and co-workers (1983)[27] detect antibodies cross-reactive with HTLV-I membrane protein in 25–30% of AIDS patients.

Gelman and co-workers (Gallo's group) (1983)[28] find evidence for presence of the viral genome of HTLV-I or an HTLV-I variant in 2 of 33 AIDS patients.

September 1983. At the Cold Spring Harbor meeting on human T-cell leukaemia–lymphoma viruses:

Montagnier and co-workers (1984)[29] report: (1) the identification of LAV-like viruses from 5 patients with lymphadenopathy and 3 patients with AIDS (homosexual, haemophiliac, Haitian); (2) the selective affinity of LAV for CD4(T4) helper lymphocytes: (3) the presence of antibodies (enzyme-linked immunosorbent assay, ELISA) against the main LAV antigens in patients with lymphadenopathy-associated syndrome (LAS) (63%) and AIDS (20%); (4) that LAV is morphologically similar to equine infectious anaemia virus (EIAV) and different from HTLVs; and (5) the antigenic cross-reactivity between core proteins of EIAV and LAV (virus isolates from LAS patients are called LAV, and from AIDS patients are called IDAV).

Gallo and co-workers (1984)[30] report the presence of HTLV-I antibodies in 10% of AIDS patients and isolates of HTLV-I or HTLV-II or variants of it in fewer than 10% of such cases.

March–April 1984. Montagnier et al. (1984)[31] by using more sera of horses infected with EIAV confirm cross-reactivity of the core proteins of LAV with that of EIAV and identify a second viral protein, p18. Vilmer, Chermann, Montagnier and co-workers (1984)[32] confirm previous isolation of an LAV-like virus from one haemophiliac and isolate another one from his asymptomatic brother.

May 1984. Gallo's group (1984) reports: (1) mass and continuous production in a clone of a permanent cell line (H9) of HTLV-III from two AIDS patients and four additional isolates (SN, BK, CS, WT) also infectious for another clone (H4) derived from the same parental cell line (Popovic, Sarngadharan, Gallo and co-workers[33]).

(2) 48 virus isolations, that is, 18 of 21 patients with pre-AIDS, 3 of 4 clinically normal mothers of juveniles with AIDS, 26 of 72 juveniles and adults with AIDS, 1 of 22 healthy male homosexuals, and 0 of 115 heterosexual subjects (Gallo, Salahuddin, Popovic and colleagues[34]). The use of anti-p24 hyperimmune sera proves that the 48 isolates belong to the same kind of virus;

(3) The introduction of the Western blot technique for clinical detection of antibodies in 88% of 48 patients with AIDS, 79% of 14 homosexuals with pre-AIDS and less than 1% of hundreds of heterosexuals. A gp41 is identified as a major viral antigen (Sarngadharan, Popovic, Gallo and co-workers[35]). Later, it is demonstrated by Veronese, Sarngadharan and Gallo to be the HTLV-III viral transmembrane component of the envelope[63].

(4) Partial characterization of the immunologically reactive proteins by the Western blot technique. (Schupbach, Sarngadharan, Popovic, Gallo and co-workers[36]).

June 1984. Safai, Gallo, Popovic and Sarngadharan report 34 of 34 (100%) of AIDS patients positive for HTLV-III antibodies, 16 of 19 (84%) of LAS patients and 0 of 14 (0%) of controls (1984)[37].

Brun-Vezinet, Barre-Sinoussi, Montagnier, Chermann and co-workers (1984)[38] publish detection of antibodies against LAV proteins by ELISA in 74.5% of the patients presenting with lymphadenopathy syndrome, 37.5% of patients with frank AIDS, 18% of healthy homosexuals, 1% of blood donors.

July 1984. Kalyanaraman, Montagnier, Francis and co-workers (1984)[40] report the detection of anti-p25 (LAV) antibodies in 51 of 125 (41%) of AIDS patients, 81 of 113 (72%) of LAS patients, and 0 of 70 of healthy individuals; Montagnier and co-workers (1984)[41] report the growth of LAV in continuous B-cell lines, most of them transformed by Epstein–Barr virus.

Klatzmann, Gluckman, Chermann, Montagnier and co-workers (1984)[42] publish: (1) the selective isolation of LAV from CD4$^+$ (T4$^+$) lymphocytes of a healthy carrier of the virus; (2) the inhibition of CD4 cell growth at the same time of *in vitro* virus production; (3) the simultaneous disappearance of the CD4 antigen at the surface of the infected CD4 lymphocytes. **August 1984.** A third group, Levy *et al.*, (1984)[43] isolate virus antigenically and structurally related to LAV from San Francisco AIDS patients.

September 1984. Cheinsong-Popov, Weiss and collaborators publish identical prevalence of antibodies against antigens of HTLV-III grown in H9 line and of LAV-1 grown in CEM line in UK patients with AIDS or at risk of AIDS (1984)[44].

Goedert, Gallo and co-workers (1984)[45] report that in a cohort of homosexual men at risk of AIDS, 53% were antibody-positive for HTLV-III. In HTLV-III antibody positive subjects, AIDS developed at 6.9% per year.

October 1984. Brun-Vezinet, Montagnier, Piot, Quinn and co-workers (1984)[46] publish the presence of antibody against LAV in 35 of 37 Zaïrean patients with AIDS.

Zagury, Gallo and co-workers (1984)[47] isolate HTLV-III from cells cultured from semen of two patients with AIDS.

November 1984. Hahn, Gallo and co-workers (1984)[48] report the molecular cloning of HTLV-III virus.

Kitchen, Allan, Essex and co-workers (1984)[49], (1985)[50] identify the viral external glycoprotein gp120, a finding confirmed by Montagnier and co-workers (1985)[51].

December 1984. Alizon, Barre-Sinoussi, Wain-Hobson, Montagnier and co-workers (1984)[52] report the molecular cloning of LAV-1.

Wong-Staal, Shaw, Gallo and co-workers (1984)[53] discover genomic heterogeneity of HTLV-III.

Dagleish, Weiss and co-workers (1984)[54] and independently Klatzmann, Gluckman, Montagnier and co-workers (1984)[55] show the CD4 molecule is involved in the receptor to the virus.

Popovic, Read-Connole and Gallo (1984)[56] publish a series of CD4-positive human neoplastic cell lines susceptible to and permissive for HTLV-III, including HUT78, Molt3 and CEM cell lines.

January 1985. The nucleotide sequence of the AIDS virus genome is established independently at the Pasteur Institute (1985)[57], at the NCI/NIH (1985)[58], at Genentech, Inc. (1985)[59] and at Chiron (1985)[60], revealing the similarity of the various isolates.

Sodroski, Wong-Staal, Gallo, Haseltine and co-workers (1985)[61] demonstrate transactivation of transcription in HTLV-III infected cells.

Shaw, Gallo and co-workers (1985)[62] discover the presence of virus in the brain.

March 1985. Redfield, Gallo and co-workers (1985)[64] describe heterosexual transmission of HTLV-III.

We wish to acknowledge with gratitude the generous help of many of our colleagues in the preparation of this history. We cannot individually thank them all here, but would like to offer special thanks to Dr. Jonas Salk for his help and guidance in completing this project.

Notes

1. Temin, H.M. & Mizutani, S. *Nature* 226, 1211–1213 (1970).
2. Baltimore, D. *Nature* 226, 1209–1211 (1970).
3. Hill, M. & Hillova, J. *C.r. Acad. Sci. Paris* 272D, 3094 (1971).
4. Montagnier, L. & Vigier, P. *C.r. Acad. Sci. Paris* 274D, 1977–1980 (1972).
5. Svoboda, I, *et al. J. gen. Virol.* 21, 47–55 (1973).
6. Spiegelman, S, *et al. Nature* 237, 1029–1031 (1970).
7. Gallo, R.C. *Nature* 234, 194–198 (1971).
8. Sarngadharan, M.G., Sarin, P.S., Reitz, M.S. & Gallo, R.C. *Nature new Biol.* 240 67–72 (1972).
9. Gerwin, B.I. & Hilstein, J.B. *Proc. natn. Acad. Sci. U.S.A.* 69, 2599–2603 (1972).
10. Morgan, D.A., Ruscatti, F.W. & Gallo, R.C. *Science* 193, 1007–1008 (1976).
11. Barre-Sinoussi, F. *et al. Ann. Microbiol.* (*Inst. Pasteur*) 130B, 349–362 (1979).
12. Poiesz, B.J. *et al. Proc. natn. Acad. Sci. U.S.A.* TT, 7415–7419 (1980).
13. Rbo, H.M. *et al. Virology* 112, 355–360 (1981); Reitz, M.S. Jr *et al. Proc. natn. Acad. Sci. U.S.A.* 78, 1887–1891. (1981); Kalyanaraman, V.S. *et al. Nature* 294, 271–273 (1981); Robert-Guroff, M. *et al. J. exp. Med.* 154, 1957–1964 (1981).
14. Hinuma, Y. *et al. Proc. natn. Acad. Sci. U.S.A.* 78, 6476–6480 (1981).
15. Yoshida, M., Miyoshi, I. & Hinuma, Y. *Proc. natn. Acad. Sci. U.S.A.* 79, 2031–2035 (1983).
16. Popovic, M. *et al. Nature* 306, 63-66 (1982).
17. Catovsky, D. *et al. Lancet* i, 639-642 (1982).
18. Blattner, W.A. *et al. Ins. J. Cancer* 30, 257–264 (1982).
19. Kalyanaraman, V.S. *et al. Science* 218, 571–575 (1982).

20. Gottlieb, M.S. *et al. Morbid. Mortal. weekly Rep.* 30, 250–252 (1981); Gottlieb, M.S. *et al. N. Engl. J. Med.* 305, 1423–1431 (1981).
21. Friedman-Kien, S.M. *et al. Morbid. Mortal. weekly Rep.* 30, 305–308 (1981).
22. Siegel, P.P. *et al. N. Engl. J. Med.* 306, 1439–1444 (1981).
23. Masur, H. *et al. N. Engl. J. Med.* 305, 1431–1438 (1981).
24. Mildvan, D. *et al. Morbid. Mortal. weekly Rep.* 31, 249–251 (1982).
25. Centers for Disease Control Task Force on Kaposi's Sarcoma and Opportunistic Infections *N. Engl. J. Med.* 306, 1248–1252 (1982).
26. Barre-Sinoussi, F. *et al. Science* 220, 868–871 (1983).
27. Essex, M. *et al. Science* 220, 859–862 (1983).
28. Gelman, E.P. *et al. Science* 220, 862–865 (1983).
29. Montagnier, L. *et al.* in *Human T-cell Leukaemia Lymphoma Viruses* (eds Gallo, R.C., Essex, M.E. & Gross, L.) 363–379 (Cold Spring Harbor Laboratory, New York, 1984).
30. Robert-Guroff, M. *et al.* in *Human T-Cell Leukaemia Lymphoma Viruses* (eds Gallo, R.C., Essex, M.E. & Gross, L.) 363–379 (Cold Spring Harbor Laboratory, New York, 1984).
31. Montagnier, L. *et al. Ann. Virol. (Inst Pasteur)* 186E. 119–134 (1984).
32. Vilmer, E. *et al. Lancet* i 753–757 (1984).
33. Popovic, M., Sarngadharan, M.Q., Read, E. & Gallo, R.C. *Science* 224, 497–500 (1984).
34. Gallo, R.C. *et al. Science* 224, 500–503 (1984).
35. Sarngadharan, M.G., Popovic, M., Bruch. L., Schupbach, J. & Gallo, R.C. *Science* 224, 506–508 (1984).
36. Schupbach, J. *et al. Science* 224, 503–505 (1984).
37. Safat, B. *et al. Lancet* i, 1435–1440 (1984).
38. Brun-Vezinet, F. *et al. Lancet* i 1253–1256 (1984).
39. Deleted.
40. Kalyanaraman, V.S. *et al, Science* 225, 321–323 (1984).
41. Montagnier, L. *Science* 226, 63–66 (1984).
42. Klatzmann, D. *et al. Science* 225, 59–69 (1984).
43. Levy, J.A. *et al. Science* 225, 840–842 (1984).
44. Cheinsong-Popov, R. *et al. Lancet* ii, 477–480 (1984).
45. Goedert, J.J. *et al. Lancet* ii, 711–716 (1984).
46. Brun-Vezinet, F. *et al. Science* 226, 453–456 (1984).
47. Zagury, D. *et al. Science* 226, 449–451 (1984).
48. Hahn, B.H. *et al. Nature* 312, 166–169 (1984).
49. Kitchen, L.W. *et al. Nature* 312, 367–369 (1984).
50. Allan, J. *et al. Science* 226, 1091–1094 (1985).
51. Montagnier, L. *et al. Virology* 144, 283–289 (1985).
52. Alizon, M. *et al. Nature* 312, 757–760 (1984).
53. Wong-Staal, F. *et al. Science* 227, 759–762 (1985).
54. Dagleish, A.G. *et al. Nature* 312, 763–767 (1984).
55. Klatzmann, D. *et al. Nature* 312, 767–768 (1984).
56. Popovic, M., Read-Connole, E. & Gallo, R.C. *Lancet* ii, 1472–1473 (1984).
57. Wain-Hobson, S., Sonigo, P., Danos, O., Cole, S. & Alizon, M. *Cell* 40, 9–17 (1985).
58. Ratner, L., Gallo, R.C. & Wong-Staal, F. *Nature* 313, 636–637 (1985).

59. Hausing, M.A. *et al. Nature* 313, 460–468 (1985).
60. Sanchez-Pescador, R. *et al. Science* 227, 484–492 (1985).
61. Sodroski, J. *et al. Science* 227, 171–173 (1985).
62. Shaw, G.M. *et al. Science* 227, 177–182 (1985).
63. Veronese, F. *et al. Science* 229, 1402–1405 (1985).
64. Redfield, R.R. *et al. J. Am. med. Ass.* 253, 1571–1573 (1985).

U.S. Public and Private Sector Resources for Fighting AIDS

Public Sector

Federal

NATIONAL SCIENCE FOUNDATION

U.S. DEPARTMENT OF DEFENSE

U.S. Army Medical Research and Development Command
  Walter Reed Army Institute of Research
    U.S. Army Medical Research Institute for Infectious Diseases

U.S. DEPARTMENT OF EDUCATION

U.S. DEPARTMENT OF HEALTH AND HUMAN SERVICES

Health Care Financing Administration
Public Health Service/Office of the Assistant Secretary for Health
  Alcohol, Drug Abuse, and Mental Health Administration
  Centers for Disease Control
  Food and Drug Administration
  Health Resources and Services Administration
National Center for Health Services Research and Health Care
    Technology Assessment
National Institutes of Health
  National Cancer Institute
  National Heart, Lung, and Blood Institute
  National Institute of Allergy and Infectious Diseases

U.S. DEPARTMENT OF STATE

Agency for International Development

This list appeared in Institute of Medicine, "Confronting AIDS: Directions for Public Health, Health Care, and Research" (Washington, D.C.: National Academy of Sciences Press, 1986).

State, City, and Local Authorities

Public health agencies (including research laboratories and education boards)
State legislatures (through policymaking and funding of research and prevention efforts)

Private Sector

Commercial Entities

Mass media
   Electronic (e.g., radio, television)
   Print (e.g., newspapers, magazines, advertising)
Pharmaceutical companies, both major and new biotechnology-based (research and development on drugs and vaccines)
Various commercial concerns (through employee education or volunteer services)

Noncommercial Organizations

Community action/volunteer groups (education/support)
National organizations
Philanthropic foundations (funding of biomedical or health services research)
Universities and other nonfederal researchers

Interviews

The following people were interviewed in person or by telephone during the preparation of this book between January 1954 and December 1986. Affiliations listed are those at the time of consultation.

Dennis Altman	La Nube University, Australia
Lawrence Altman	*New York Times*
Virginia Apuzzo	National Gay Task Force
Peter Arno	University of California, San Francisco
François Barre-Sinoussi	Pasteur Institute
Donald Berreth	CDC
Jeremy Bishop	*Wall Street Journal*
Edward N. Brandt, Jr.	Chancellor, University of Maryland at Baltimore
Brett Cassens	American Association for Human Rights
William Check	Journalist
James Curran	CDC
Marcus Conant	University of California, San Francisco
Jean-Claude Chermann	Pasteur Institute
Walter Dowdle	CDC
Donald Drake	*Philadelphia Enquirer*

Anthony Fauci	NIAID
Donald Francis	CDC
Peter Fischinger	NCI
Alvin Friedman-Kien	New York University
James Hill	NIAID
Mathilde Krim	AMFAR
Martin Landry	GAO
Lewis Lapham	*Harper's* magazine
Philip Lee	University of California, San Francisco
Arthur Levine	NICHHD
Jay Levy	University of California, San Francisco General Hospital
Luc Montagnier	Pasteur Institute
John La Montaigne	NIAID
Malcolm Martin	NIAID
James Mason	CDC
Jay E. Menitove	South Western Wisconsin Blood Center
Stephen Meskin	HCFA
Lawrence Mass	Physician and journalist
Maureen Myers	NIAID
Frank Polk	Johns Hopkins University
Olivia Preble	Uniformed Services, University of the Health Sciences
Frederick Robbins	President, Institute of Medicine
Wilmon Rushing	CDC
Gerald Sandler	American Red Cross
Kenneth Sell	NIAID
David Sencer	Director, New York Public Health Service
Mervyn Silverman	Director, San Francisco Public Health Department

Ralph Sonnabend	Physician
Susan Steinmetz	Staff member, Subcommittee of Intergovernmental Relations, U.S. House of Representatives
Samuel Thier	President, Institute of Medicine
Paul Volberding	San Francisco General Hospital
Timothy Westmoreland	Counsel, Staff of Henry Waxman, U.S. House of Representatives

Notes

Introduction

1. Dr. Halfan Mahler, in announcing a massive international effort to combat AIDS on November 20, 1986, as quoted in The *New York Times,* November 20, 1986, p. 1.

1. The Advent of AIDS

1. From a tape-recorded recollection of early findings about AIDS, made in 1982 by Dr. Friedman-Kien and provided by him.
2. The figures were provided by Wilmon Rushing of the CDC AIDS Activity during an interview in Atlanta on April 18, 1985.
3. From Levine's presentation at the annual meeting of the American Association for the Advancement of Science in May 1984.
4. "Follow-up on Kaposi's sarcoma and pnemocystis pneumonia," *MMWR,* 30 (August 28, 1981), pp. 409–410.
5. In characteristically understated terms, the *MMWR* of July 16, 1982, noted: "The clinical and immunologic features these three patients share are strikingly similar to those observed among certain individuals from the following groups: homosexual males, heterosexuals who abuse drugs, and Haitians who recently entered the United States. Although the cause of severe immune dysfunction is unknown, the occurrence among the three hemophiliac cases suggests the possible transmission of an agent through blood products." And although understated, the conclusion clearly showed concern and alarm: "CDC has notified directors of hemophilia centers about these cases and, with the National Hemophilia Foundation, has initiated collaborative surveillance. A Public Health Service advisory committee is being formed to consider the implication of these findings. Physicians diagnosing opportunistic infections in hemophilia patients who have not received immunosuppressive therapy are encouraged to report them to the CDC through local and state health departments."
6. "Hepatitis B Virus Vaccine Safety: Report of an Interagency group," *MMWR, 31* (September 3, 1982), pp. 465–467.
7. "Update on Acquired Immune Deficiency Syndrome" *MMWR, 31* (September 24, 1982), pp. 507–514.

8. David Talbot and Larry Bush, "At Risk, AIDS: Downplaying the Plague" *Mother Jones* (April 1985), p. 36.

9. The two papers the editorial discussed were: J. Oleske et al., "Immune Deficiency Syndrome in Children," *JAMA,* 249 (May 6, 1983), pp. 2345–2349, and A. Rubinstein et al., "Acquired Immunodeficiency with Reversed T_4/T_8 Ratios in Infants Born to Promiscuous and Drug-Addicted Mothers," ibid., pp. 2350–2356. The editorial noted: "The implications of AIDS in this patient population are several. It took some time for people to believe that AIDS was indeed transmissible. Then it was assumed that it could only be transmitted by sexual contact among homosexuals and by blood products. Recently, the CDC has reported AIDS among the female sex partners of IV drug users, and others have reported AIDS among female prostitutes. The findings of AIDS in infants and children who are household contacts of patients with AIDS or persons with risks for AIDS had enormous implications with regard to ultimate transmissibility of this syndrome. First, it is possible that AIDS can be vertically transmitted [that is, genetically, or from mother to child either in utero, or during birth]. Perhaps even more important is the possibility that routine close contact, as within a family household, can spread the disease. If, indeed, the latter is true, then AIDS takes on an entirely new dimension." Anthony S. Fauci, "The Acquired Immune Deficiency Syndrome—The Ever-Broadening Clinical Syndrome," ibid. pp. 2375–2376.

10. Fauci appeared on the Donahue show on July 13, 1983, along with Edward Brandt who observed and then retold this story.

11. See Dennis Altman, *AIDS in the Mind of America* (Garden City, N.Y.: Anchor Press, 1986) for a discussion of the views of the homosexual community.

12. From an interview with Edward Brandt, April 5, 1985.

13. Brandt was recruited in 1981 into Richard Schweiker's HHS from his position as vice chancellor for health affairs in the University of Texas system. In an administration where appropriately conservative credentials were considered a prerequisite for appointment, he appeared to have no strong ideological commitment.

14. Talbot and Bush, "At Risk, AIDS: Downplaying the Plague."

15. U.S. Bureau of the Census, 1984 population figures.

16. Dedicated AIDS units were instituted in New York in late 1985.

17. Altman, *AIDS in the Mind of America;* William A. Check, "Public Education on AIDS: Not Only the Media's Responsibility," Hastings Center Report, 4 (August 1985), pp. 27–31; Edwin Diamond and Christopher M. Bellitto, "The Great Verbal Cover-Up," *Washington Journalism Review* (March 1986), pp. 38–42; and William A. Check, "The Political Model of Reporting: Nonspecific Symptoms in Media Communications About AIDS," a background paper commissioned for the Institute of Medicine's study about AIDS, 1986.

18. Dennis Altman, in the *Village Voice,* April 2, 1985, pp. 18–20.

19. From an interview with Mervyn Silverman on January 25, 1985.

20. See articles published in the *San Francisco Chronicle* during 1984 and collected in "The Year of the Plague," a supplement of the *Chronicle.*

21. Office of Technology Assessment, U.S. Congress, "Blood Policy and Technology," #07A-H-260 (January 1985).

22. Ibid., p. 5.

23. A. G. Fettner and W. A. Check, *The Truth About AIDS* (New York: Holt, Rinehart, and Winston, 1984), p. 135.
24. Personal communication from Dr. Menitove.
25. "Federal Response to AIDS," Hearings of the House Oversight Committee on Government Operations, August 1–2, 1983, p. 167.
26. "Prevention of Acquired Immune Deficiency Syndrome (AIDS): Report of Inter-Agency Recommendations, *MMWR*, 32 (March 4, 1983), pp. 101–104.
27. The following four articles were published in *Science*, 224 (1984): M. Popovic et al., "Detection, Isolation, and Continuous Production of Cytopathic Retroviruses (HTLV-III) from Patients with AIDS and Pre-AIDS," pp. 497–500: R. C. Gallo et al., "Frequent Detection and Isolation of Cytopathic Retroviruses (HTLV-III) from Patients with AIDS and at Risk for AIDS," pp. 500–503; J. Schupbach et al., "Serological Analysis of a Subgroup of Human T-Lymphotropic Retroviruses (HTLV-III) Associated with AIDS," pp. 503–505; and M. G. Sarngadharan et al., "Antibodies Reactive with Human T-Lymphotropic Retroviruses (HTLV-III) in the Serum of Patients with AIDS," pp. 506–508.
28. F. Barre-Sinoussi et al., "Isolation of a T-Lymphotropic Retrovirus from a Patient at Risk for Acquired Immune Deficiency Syndrome (AIDS)," *Science*, 220 (1983), pp. 868–871.
29. Richard Carter, *Breakthrough—The Saga of Jonas Salk* (New York: Trident Press, 1966).
30. Sandra Panem, *The Interferon Crusade* (Washington, D.C.: Brookings Institution, 1984).
31. Edward Brandt recalled that Gallo expressed this opinion at a meeting held in Brandt's office before the press conference.
32. Dr. James Mason, quoted in an interview with Lawrence K. Altman, "Federal Official Says He Believes Cause of AIDS Has Been Found," *New York Times*, April 22, 1984.
33. For detailed discussion of the patent dispute see articles in *Science* magazine: December 16, 1983, p. 1178; November 1, 1985, p. 518; November 8, 1985, p. 640; January 3, 1986, p. 11; May 9, 1986, pp. 697 and 699; July 25, 1986, p. 414.
34. A legal battle later erupted over the provenance of the AIDS virus between the U.S. government and the Pasteur Institute. See Lawrence K. Altman for the *New York Times* throughout June, 1986; "U.S. Court Dismisses French Suit over the Discovery of AIDS," *New York Times*, July 10, 1986, p. A20; see also Deborah Barnes, "AIDS Patent Dispute Settled," *Science*, 236 (1987), p. 171; and Appendix A.
35. "The Chronology of AIDS Research," *Nature*, 326 (1987), pp. 435–436.
36. The editorial in the *New York Native*—written by Charles Ortleb and entitled "Should Gallo and Essex Be In Jail?" (No. 117, June 3–16, 1985)—said:

    "It's time that every scientist in the world with a shred of integrity began asking whether certain members of their community are up to their necks in scientific fraud. There are at least two allegations that must be resolved immediately . . .

    "Allegation #1—That Robert Gallo 'discovered' the virus Dr. Luc Montagnier of the Pasteur Institute gave to him—i.e., that Gallo's lab 'stole' the discovery from the French . . .

"Allegation #2—That the linking of an AIDS-associated virus with HTLV-I and HTLV-II [by naming it HTLV-III] was a deliberate attempt to confuse scientists and the public, to enjoy acclaim, and to obtain grants and other benefits, including public moneys . . .

"What Can You Do About It? First of all get angry, as angry as you'd get if someone had just killed your lover. Then call up every Senator, every Congressman you can get on the phone and demand an immediate investigation of Robert Gallo and 'his' virus before this fraud and this scientific standstill in fact does kill you, your lover and millions of other Americans."

37. See, for example, the series of news articles on the politics of science in AIDS in *Science*, May 4, 1984; October 25, 1985; November 1, 1985; November 29, 1985; December 6 and 20, 1985; January 3, 1986; and "Tracing the Origins of AIDS," *Newsweek* (May 7, 1984).

38. One tradition among scientists is that they must never take credit for something they have not done; another, that everyone legitimately involved in an effort should be acknowledged. This tradition is sometimes taken to comic lengths. For example, here is a July 1984 letter to the editor that appeared in the British medical journal *Lancet:*

"Sir,—I am sure that many scientists believe that the elucidation of the epidemiology, cause and pathogenesis of the acquired immune deficiency syndrome (AIDS) will advance our knowledge of immunology considerably. AIDS appeared out of the blue a few years ago and, apart from causing immunodeficiency, it has been responsible for two other syndromes—the 'minimal publishable unit syndrome' (MUPS) and the 'how many authors can I cram onto one paper syndrome' (HMACICOOPS).

"In your June 23 issue, 18 authors publish a letter stating that they are doing an experiment with 23 monkeys . . . I cannot believe that it takes 18 people to do these experiments on 23 monkeys or that 18 people in six centers can write a letter . . ."

39. James Watson, *The Double Helix* (New York: Atheneum, 1968); and Anne Sayre, *Rosalind Franklin and DNA* (New York: Norton, 1975).

40. Accounts of the origin of the Salk-Sabin dispute can be found in Saul Benison's *Tom Rivers: Reflections on a Life in Medicine and Science* (Cambridge, Mass.: MIT press, 1967), and in Richard Carter's *Breakthrough: The Saga of Jonas Salk* (New York: Trident Press, 1966).

41. Nicholas Wade, *The Nobel Duel* (New York: Doubleday, 1981).

42. It should be noted that Waxman was also a member of the Government Operations Committee, but used his Science and Technology Subcommittee as the platform for issues he wanted to explore. The Senate was less active than the House.

43. Edward N. Brandt, in an address entitled, "AIDS: The Ethical, Legal, and Social Considerations," sponsored by Public Responsibility in Medicine and Research, given on April 25, 1985, in Boston.

44. Brandt, in an address to the School of Social Work at the University of Maryland, September 1985.

45. See comments of Ted Weiss in "Federal Response to AIDS," Hearings of the

House Oversight Committee on Government Operations, August 1–2, 1983, p. 478.

46. See ibid. for details of the confrontation and copies of correspondence.

47. From an interview with Martin Landry, Washington, D.C. July 25, 1985.

48. According to the 16th edition of *American Men and Women of Science,* William Herbert Foege was a medical officer with the Lutheran Church-Missouri Synod at the Nigeria Mission in 1965–66.

49. Memorandum from HHS Secretary Margaret Heckler to Representative Ted Weiss, May 12, 1983.

50. See correspondence and documents from "Federal Response to AIDS."

51. Ibid., Ted Weiss to William Foege:

"It again becomes necessary to reiterate the subcommittee's position regarding the conduct of our oversight investigation at CDC. It is unfortunate that you are continuing to delay the subcommittee's performance of its investigation into the Federal response to the AIDS crisis.

"First, as you know, there is no legal basis for denying the subcommittee access to files maintained at the Center based either on grounds of 'budget information, policy formation, or patient confidentiality.' With regard to patient information, I reiterate that the subcommittee has no interest or intention of removing the names of patients from CDC files. However, we must maintain the ability to review files directly."

In rejoinder Foege argued in a letter to Weiss on July 25, 1983 as follows:

"Your letter, with its attached procedural recommendations, makes it clear that you do intend for your staff to see the names of patients . . . the investigation of AIDS is hampered by the concern of patients, physicians, and local health authorities that names given to CDC could not be safeguarded. Your request lends substance to that concern. We are now working on a procedure which would preclude CDC's receipt of names as part of its AIDS surveillance system. All documents would be identified by code. Such a procedure will obviously extract a price in the efficiency and effectiveness of this and subsequent investigations, but may be the only way to assure that *accurate medical information* is collected from patients who are concerned about confidentiality and exposure. Your request to see names makes it clear that we will have to pay that price in order to retain the cooperation of State and local health departments and physicians and patients. In summary, our attempts to solve the problem of AIDS will be markedly slowed by any requests for patient identification data which will undermine the accuracy or availability of future data collection.

"In the meantime, I trust you will agree that there are also moral factors involved in this instance that should transcend the legal prerogatives of Congress or the Executive Branch. These patients are already suffering under a burden of physical disintegration, social ostracism, and an unknown future. I cannot add to their burden with the possibility that they will be identified to a Congressional office."

52. See interview with Landry, note 47 above.

53. "Twenty-Ninth Report by the Committee on Government Operations, together with Dissenting Views, on the Federal Response to AIDS" (U.S. Government Printing Office, November 30, 1983).

2. Monitoring Public Health

1. John Duffy, "School Vaccination: Precursor to School Medical Inspection," *Journal of The History of Medicine and Allied Sciences,* 33 (July 1978), pp. 344–355.
2. 1 Stat. L., 605–606.
3. Jesse Steinfeld, in *Health in America: 1776–1976,* DHEW Publication no. (HRA) 76–616 (U.S. Public Health Service), pp. 68–69.
4. 16 Stat. L., 169.
5. Donald R. Whitlash, ed., *The Greenwood Encyclopedia of American Institutions: Government Agencies* (Westport, Conn.: Greenwood Press, 1983), p. 453.
6. William Shonick, "Public Health Services: Background and Present Status," in S. J. Williams and P. R. Torrens, eds., *Introduction to Health Services,* 2nd ed. (New York: John Wiley, 1984), pp. 98–101.
7. Lister Hill, in *Health in America: 1776–1976.* DHEW Publication no. (HRA) 76–616 (U.S. Public Health Service), p. 9.
8. Paul Starr, *Social Transformation of American Medicine* (New York: Basic Books, 1982), p. 184.
9. Paul R. Torrens, "Historical Evolution and Overview of Health Services," in Williams and Torrens, eds. *Introduction to Health Services,* p. 5.
10. John K. Iglehart, "Health Policy Report: The Centers for Disease Control," *NEJM,* 308 (March 10, 1983), pp. 604–608.
11. Ibid., p. 605.
12. Ibid., p. 604.
13. W. Shonick, "Public Health Services," in Williams and Torrens, eds., *Introduction,* p. 99.
14. H. Emerson, *Local Health Units for the Nation* (New York: Commonwealth Fund, 1945).
15. Vital statistics include recording, tabulation, interpretation, and publication of the essential facts of births, deaths and reportable diseases. It is the state which determines when a disease is reportable, and requires physicians to report. States also provide the service of licensure for physicians. The decentralized authority of reporting and the lack of consistent policy had been of major concern in AIDS.
16. W. Shonick, "Public Health Services," in Williams and Torrens, eds., *Introduction,* p. 109.
17. Torrens, "Historical Evolution," in Williams and Torrens, eds., *Introduction,* p. 113.

3. Biomedical Research Institutions

1. 27 Stat. L., 309.
2. Biologics Control Act of 1902, 32 Stat. L., 712.
3. The Food, Drug, and Insecticide Administration was created in 1927 and subsequently renamed the Food and Drug Administration.
4. Donald R. Whitlash, ed., *The Greenwood Encyclopedia of American Institutions: Government Agencies* (Westport, Conn.: Greenwood Press, 1983), pp. 251–257.

5. Vernon Lippard, *A Half-Century of American Medical Education, 1920–1970* (New York: Josiah Macy Jr. Foundation, 1974), p. 22.

6. Ibid.

7. NCI-enabling legislation was the National Cancer Act of 1937.

8. Hill-Burton Act, 1946 (P.L. 79–725); the Hospital Survey and Construction Act.

9. Grants-in-aid (or intergovernmental grants) are funds made available by the federal government to state and local governments. There are great differences in state fiscal resources as well as in the relative burden of a public health problem; compare, for example, the numbers of AIDS patients in New York and San Francisco with other American cities. Because these fiscal, demographic, and other discrepancies exist, and because most health problems do not have a purely local effect, federal grants-in-aid can work to spread the fiscal burden of health care and provide leverage for the federal government to affect state and local policies.

   A grant-in-aid may be a general or block grant which is available for any type of expenditure. Alternatively, selective grants, such as categorical program or individual project grants, are tied to specific uses. Grants may be "matching grants," calculated as the same proportion of the recipients total expenditure, or may be "nonmatching grants," which are not tied to the recipients' other resources. Each of these kinds of grants-in-aid may be used for medical research.

10. The research strategy required an effort to understand the natural history of the disease, a delienation of the different types of polio virus, the development of animal models for research, and models for vaccination. For a detailed description of the National Foundation's "Eleven Point" Program, see Saul Benison, *Tom Rivers: A Life in Medicine and Science* (Cambridge, Mass.: MIT Press, 1967), pp. 229–233. Federal participation in the NFIP-initiated effort came only in the 1950s, after an experimental vaccine had been developed.

11. Office of Management and Budget, *Historical Tables, Budget of the U.S. Government, FY 1986* (Washington, D.C.: U.S. Government Printing Office, 1986), Table 10.2.

12. The institutes are: Allergy and Infectious Diseases; Arthritis, Diabetes, and Kidney Disease; Cancer; Child Health and Human Development; Dental Research; Environmental Health Sciences; Eye; General Medical Sciences; Heart, Lung, and Blood; Aging; and Neurological and Communicative Disorders and Stroke.

13. Institute of Medicine, *Responding to Needs and Scientific Opportunity: The Organizational Structure of the National Institutes of Health* (Washington, D.C.: National Academy Press, 1984).

14. The IOM, National Academy of Science, and National Academy of Engineering are associated with the National Research Council. All operate under a charter from Congress.

15. Michael A. Stoto and James D. Ebert, "The Organizational Structure of NIH," *NEJM*, 312 (June 1985), pp. 1634–1637.

16. Ibid.

17. Extramural activities are organized in individual institutes, in the more centralized Division of Research Grants (DRG), in the Division of Research Resources (DRR), and in the Fogarty International Center (FIC).

18. Estimates are based on figures in the NIH *Fact Book,* NIH Publication no. 85–1261, June 1985.

19. Donald Fredrickson, NIH director from 1974 through 1982, reinforced this symbolism by making the number of RO1s granted each year a political platform for the continuity of medical research. Some pundits feel that when Fredrickson tried to establish a minimum acceptable level of research grants, he established a "ceiling" rather than a "floor." Nevertheless, in the 1980s, debate about the federal government's commitment to a particular area of research most often centered on how many RO1 grants were supporting the area. This extended to health research in general: for example, when the 1986 reauthorization came under consideration. At that time, a discussion between the Congress and OMB centered on whether 5,000, 6,000, or 6,500 new and competing RO1s would be funded. Congress wanted to fund 6,500 grants, OMB wanted 5,000, and a deal was struck for approximately 6,200.

20. Codified criteria govern the selection of reviewers, conflict of interest, and other concerns for the peer review process. One example of such criteria can be found in the "Peer Review of Contract Proposals at the NCI, Information for Contract Proposal Reviewers," June 1981. Within the research establishment, service on a peer review panel carries prestige and is often seen as an essential step in career development. The study sections are charged with the technical review of proposals. Section members are supposed to base their ratings strictly on the perceived contribution of the proposed research to the growth of knowledge in the relevant area. Study sections review proposals of diverse institutes. This indicates the overlapping nature of technical expertise the various institutes rely on.

21. Traditionally, peer review of intramural research has been organized ad hoc and through the scientific director's office. In the last ten years demands for greater scientific accountability resulted in a more formalized review of intramural programs through the Board of Scientific Advisers (composed of extramural scientists). Unlike the statutory requirement for each institute's National Advisory Council (a group of advisers outside NIH) to review all extramural grants for relevancy to their institute's mission, the use of advisory boards in establishing the direction of intramural programs is not mandated by law, but is established through NIH policy. In recognition of these differences, a 1984 IOM study of the structure of NIH questioned whether the same standards of external review employed by extramural programs should be extended to intramural programs.

22. Dr. Thomas Rivers played a prominent role in managing the targeted research effort that the National Foundation mounted to develop a polio vaccine in the late 1930s. He recalled that: "During the first year of the Foundation's existence, the Scientific Research Committee received any number of applications for grants from individual investigators and, while many were worthwhile in themselves, together they did not seem to be going anywhere. They were too haphazard for a program and I thought that the Foundation would be better served if a committee surveyed the field of polio research and blocked out problems that needed solution. With such a guide in hand, I felt that the committee should seek out the men and institutions capable of researching such problems and support them with grants." See Benison, *Tom Rivers* p. 231.

In answer to Benison's query about whether there was opposition to a targeted approach to polio research, Rivers replied: "Indeed there was. Several members of the committee didn't like my idea, among them George McCoy and Charles Armstrong. They felt that the Foundation would be better advised if it simply continued to give grants to competent investigators of accredited institutions who voluntarily expressed their wish to do research into the causes and prevention of polio" (ibid., p. 232).

23. P.L. 88–164.
24. P.L. 89–793.
25. P.L. 91–616.
26. P.L. 92–255.
27. P.L. 93–282.
28. The Robert Wood Johnson Foundation initiated a program to fund AIDS-related services in 1986.

4. Delivering Health Care

1. Paul. R. Torrens, "Historical Evolution and Overview of Health Services," in S. J. Williams and P. R. Torrens, eds., *Introduction to Health Services*, 2nd ed. (New York: John Wiley, 1984), p. 14.
2. F. A. Wilson and D. Newhauser, *Health Services in the United States* (Cambridge, Mass.: Ballinger, 1982), p. 2.
3. Nancy Milo, *Primary Care and the Public's Health* (Lexington, Mass.: Lexington Books, 1983), p. 21.
4. HCFA, Office of Financial and Actuarial Analysis, Division of National Cost Estimates. Cited in the *HCFA Review*, 6-3 (Spring 1985).
5. P. R. Lee, "AIDS: Allocating Resources for Research and Patient Care," *Issues in Science and Technology*, 2 (Winter 1986), pp. 66–73.
6. Congressional testimony of Paul Volberding, director, AIDS Activity of San Francisco General Hospital, on July 1985.
7. In late 1986 the drug AZT (azidothymidine) was found to be useful in treating (but not curing) AIDS. Despite increasing use, throughout 1987 AZT treatment was still in the process of being evaluated for efficacy and safety under varying clinical circumstances.
8. "Sec.2.(a)(3). The many and increasing responses to these [health] problems by the public sector (Federal, State, and local) and the private sector have not resulted in a comprehensive, rational approach to the present—
    (A) lack of uniformly effective methods of delivering health care;
    (B) maldistribution of health care facilities and manpower; and;
    (C) increasing costs of health care.
    (b) In recognition of the magnitude of the problems described . . . and the urgency placed on their solution, it is the purpose of this Act to facilitate the development of recommendations for a national health planning policy, to augment areawide and State planning for health services, manpower, and facilities, and to authorize financial assistance for the development of resources to further that policy."
    From the National Health Planning and Resources Development Act, 1974, P.L. 93–641.
9. P.L. 98–49.
10. July 21, 1930; P.L. 71–536, Veterans Affairs Consolidation Act. According to

Jesse Steinfeld, "The Public Health Service played a significant role [in addressing military health needs] in World War I. It moved beyond sanitation around military camps and in civilian areas and invested more resources in health care for Federal beneficiaries at Public Health Service hospitals and in the manufacture of needed vaccines and sera as well as research regarding others still to come. The Public Health Service began a vigorous venereal disease campaign during the war and also a large-scale, effective malaria control campaign . . . The Public Health Service in 1920 had not only the Marine Hospitals but also the responsibility for hospital care of the discharged veterans of World War I. Dr. Claude Lavender was in charge of the multiple veterans programs as 'Assistant Surgeon General in Charge of Marine Hospitals and Relief.' Soon, however, Secretary of the Treasury Andrew Mellon transferred from the Public Health Service to the Treasury's War Risk Insurance Bureau the responsibility for giving medical examinations to determine a veteran's disability rating and compensation. This left only inpatient and outpatient medical care to the Public Health Service. Within six months, the re-named Veterans Bureau became independent of the Treasury Department, reporting directly to the President. The Bureau, however, held on to its Public Health Service legacy: 57 hospitals, 13,000 patients, 17,000 beds, 900 physicians and dentists, 1,400 nurses, and 9 new hospitals still under construction. Dr. Lavender's Public Health Service hospital division was left with 24 Marine hospitals and 3,000 beds. (One measure of the storm created by establishment of the Veterans Bureau: its first chief resigned under fire, was indicted, prosecuted, and sent to prison.) The Public Health Service and Veterans Administration have continued as separate systems to this day, although the bitterness of the 1922 split has disappeared. Yet the problems of coordinating appropriate V.A. and PHS activities remain." Jesse Steinfeld, in *Health in America: 1776–1976*, DHEW Publication no. (HRA) 76–616 (U.S. Public Health Service), pp. 72–73.

11. Mervyn F. Silverman and Deborah B. Silverman, "AIDS and the Threat to Public Health," *The Hastings Report* (August 1985). Special supplement, pp. 19–22.

12. Kathleen Teltsch, "Foundations Widen Efforts in AIDS," *New York Times*, July 28, 1987, p. B18.

13. This bill, H.R. 5438, read: ". . . given the diversity of federal health programs which range from research conducted by or through the NIH to the administrations of the programs under titles XVIII and XIX of the Social Security Act by the Health Care Financing Administration, there is a need for an Undersecretary for Health to serve as a single management focus."

14. Marlene Cimons, "OMB Would Give Surgeon General Command of Fight Against AIDS," *Washington Post*, January 2, 1986.

5. Economics and Politics

1. These and subsequent figures are derived from the U.S. Department of Commerce, Bureau of the Census, *Statistical Abstract of the United States, 1986;* from the *Budget of the United States, FY1986;* and *Historical Tables, Budget of the United States Government, 1986* (Washington, D.C.: U.S. Government Printing Office, 1986).

2. OMB and CBO can be viewed as competing analytic teams. The magnitude of their enterprise is staggering. In FY83 OMB claimed 611 employees and CBO, 220. For the OMB figures, see the Statistical Abstract of the United States, 1986. The CBO figure was provided by Alice Rivlin in a personal communication with the author, November 1985.

3. P.L. 93–344, Congressional Budget and Impoundment Control Act of 1974, and the Budget and Accounting Act of 1921.

4. From hearings of the Oversight subcommittee of the House Committee on Government Operations, the U.S. House of Representatives, 98th Congress, August 1 and 2, 1983.

5. William Shonick, "Public Health Services: Background and Present Status," in S. J. Williams and Paul R. Torrens, eds., Introduction to Health Services, 2nd ed. (New York: John Wiley, 1984).

6. From hearings of the Oversight Subcommittee, August 1 and 2, 1983. Sencer was commissioner of health for the city of New York; Silverman was director of public health for the city of San Francisco.

7. See "Preventive Health Amendments of 1984," H.R. 5538.

8. From an interview with Mervyn Silverman, January 25, 1985.

9. OMB Circular No. A–10, "Responsibility for Disclosure with Respect to the Budget," revised November 12, 1976. The policies stated in this document were in force during the initial period of the AIDS epidemic. These policies were superseded by OMB Circular No. A–11, June 25, 1985.

10. Lee made this comment at the annual meeting of the IOM, National Academy of Sciences, October 16, 1985. See also Issues in Science and Technology (Winter 1985), pp. 66–73.

11. These figures are presented as current dollars.

12. Appropriations bill for the Departments of Labor and Health and Human Services for FY85, enacted November 1986.

13. Timothy Westmoreland, personal communication, February 1986.

6. Unique Elements

1. Office of Technology Assessment, Review of the Public Health Service's Response to AIDS (Washington, D.C., U.S. Congress, OTA-TM-H-24, February 1985).

2. See David Talbot and Lawrence Bush, "At Risk," Mother Jones, 10–111 (April 1985), pp. 28–37; David Black, The Plague Years (New York: Simon and Schuster, 1986); and Charles Ortleb, "Should Gallo and Essex Be in Jail," editorial in the New York Native, 117 (June 3–6, 1985).

3. H.R. 2713 (subsequently P.L. 98–49, Public Health Service Amendment, 97 Stat. 245) was enacted in July 1983.

4. In "Hearings before the Subcommittee on Health and the Environment of the Committee on Energy and Commerce," House of Representatives, 98th Congress, 1st sess. on Public Health Emergency Act-H.R. 2713, May 9, 1983 (GAO, 1983), p. 7.

5. Ibid., p. 17.

6. Ibid., pp. 17–18.

7. Edward N. Brandt, Jr., "Executive Task Force on AIDS," Memorandum to Public Health Service Heads, May 7, 1984.

8. Edward N. Brandt, Jr., "Proposed FY84 Supplemental and FY85 Amendment for Acquired Immune Deficiency Syndrome," Memorandum to the Secretary of Health and Human Services, May 1984.
9. Virginia Apuzzo, personal communication, December 1985.
10. See Arthur M. Silverstein, *Pure Politics, Impure Science: The Swine Flu Affair* (Baltimore, Md.: Johns Hopkins University Press, 1981).
11. "Twenty-ninth Report by the Committee on Government Operations, together with Dissenting Views, on the Federal Response to AIDS" (U.S. Government Printing Office, November 30, 1983), pp. 22, 26.
12. Colin Norman, "News and Comment: A Plea for Academia," *Science*, 231 (January 31, 1986), p. 447.
13. Arthur S. Levine, in a symposium, "AIDS: Can Research Be Mobilized in Response to an Emergency?" at the American Association for the Advancement of Science annual meeting, May 31, 1984, New York.
14. James Curran, in the same symposium.
15. Executive Office of the President, Office of Management and Budget, *"Major Policy Initiatives: Fiscal Year 1987,"* p. 22.
16. From hearings of the Oversight Subcommittee of the House Committee on Government Operations, August 1 and 2, 1983, p. 166.
17. From Brett Cassens' comments at the annual meeting of the American Public Health Association, Washington, D.C., November 18, 1985.
18. Stephen Meskin, Chief Medicaid Actuary, DHHS, HCFA, personal communication, November 1985.

7. Who's in Charge?

1. Most congressional testimony developed by executive branch offices is cleared through OMB. Concerning budgetary matters, OMB Circular A-10 stated: "4. *Agency testimony before and communications with Congress on budgetary matters.* In furnishing information on appropriations and budgetary matters, representatives of agencies should be aware of the limitations on such communications, including the limitation that: 'No estimate or request for an appropriation and no request for an increase in an item of any such estimate or request . . . shall be submitted to Congress or any committee thereof by any officer or employee of any department or establishment, unless at the request of either House or Congress' (31 U.S.C. 15). Furthermore, agency representatives should be aware of restrictions upon communications to influence legislation that are not conducted through proper official channels (18 U.S.C. 1913)."

   This policy was made even more explicit by Circular A-11 in 1985. OMB's "Analysis of Changes" accompanying Circular A-11 stated: "This subsection (11.9) has been expanded to consolidate guidance on responsibilities for disclosure with respect to the budget. Included is a new requirement for OMB clearance of oversight testimony that affects budget matters."
2. Public Health Service, "AIDS Operational Plan" (Fall 1984), pp. 6–7.
3. In the summer of 1985, the military implemented HTLV-III antibody screening of all personnel. Private insurance companies considered antibody testing as a

criteria for eligibility for coverage, and discussions of screening food handlers, teachers, and others abounded.

4. See PHS, "AIDS Operational Plan," pp. 15–16: "Initially, coordination of PHS AIDS activities was effectively accomplished under the direct supervision of the Assistant Secretary for Health (ASH) through a PHS Executive Committee composed of members from all PHS agencies involved in AIDS research and public health activity . . . With revised and accelerated activities generated by the discovery of HTLV-III in April 1984, the coordinating mechanism was modified to provide for an Executive Task Force in lieu of the Committee and with specific work panels on resources, science affairs and public information and education. Chairpersons of the panels are on the Task Force in addition to heads of agencies. The Panels include appropriate program experts from a cross section of agencies and at various levels."

5. Between 1981 and 1984 the attempt by Congress to legislate more detailed accountability of research programming failed. In November 1985, at the eleventh hour, President Reagan vetoed the 1986 NIH reauthorization bill on the grounds that Congress had imposed too close oversight over the agency's operations. Within the next two weeks, the Congress overwhelmingly overturned his veto.

6. Timothy Westmoreland, in comments during a panel discussion at "AIDS: Public Policy Dimensions," a forum convened by the United Hospital Fund of New York, New York City (January 16–17, 1986).

7. The IOM was chartered in 1970 by the National Academy of Sciences to enlist distinguished members of the appropriate professions in the examination of policy matters pertaining to public health. The institute acts under the Academy's 1863 congressional charter responsibility to be an adviser to the federal government, but uses its own initiative in identifying issues of medical care, research, and education.

8. For a discussion of the political aspects of the National Academy of Sciences, see Philip M. Boffey, *The Brain Bank of America: An Inquiry into the Politics of Science* (New York: McGraw Hill, 1975).

9. OTA report, "Review of the Public Health Service's Response to AIDS" (February 1985).

10. From interviews with Frederick Robbins and Edward N. Brandt, 1984 and 1985.

11. "Twenty-Ninth Report by the Committee on Government Operations, together with Dissenting Views, on the Federal Response to AIDS" (Washington, D.C.: U.S. Government Printing Office, November 30, 1983).

8. The Flow of Information

1. Arnold S. Relman, editor of the *NEJM*, commenting on his decision to expedite publication of articles about AIDS, has noted: "By the end of 1981, after publication of the initial reports, material on AIDS began arriving at the *New England Journal of Medicine*'s editorial office in a swelling stream. Now, after nearly four years [1985], hardly a week passes without the receipt of at least several manuscripts and a handful of letters. Because of the intense interest and

the need to disseminate reliable new information as quickly as possible, we have been giving manuscripts about AIDS special treatment. We expedite the peer review process and, once a paper has been accepted, we allow the authors publicly to disclose their results even before the date of publication, if they wish to do so. Furthermore, in certain cases we are prepared to suspend our so-called 'Ingelfinger Rule,' which ordinarily prohibits consideration of material that has had prior public dissemination." See Arnold S. Relman, "AIDS: The Emerging Ethical Dilemmas," Hastings Center Report, Special Supplement (August 1985), pp. 1–2.

2. From Colin Norman, "AIDS Virology: A Battle on Many Fronts," *Science*, 230 (November 1985), p. 519.
3. Ann G. Fettner and William Check, *The Truth About AIDS* (New York: Holt, Rinehart and Winston, 1984).
4. Ibid, p. 97.
5. From interview with Frederick Robbins, December 15, 1984.
6. See discussion of patent dispute in Chapter 1.
7. Scheduled for presentation were remarks from Abbott Laboratories, Cellular Products, Centocor, E. I. DuPont de Nemours & Co., Electronucleonics, Genetic Systems, Litton Industries, Ortho Diagnostics, and Travenol/Genentech Diagnostics.
8. See, for example, Sandra G. Boodman, "Views of Four U.S. AIDS Panelists Hit," *Washington Post*, August 26, 1987, p. Al.

9. Communicating with the Public

1. Institute for Health Policy Analysis, "AIDS: A Case Study in Health Risk Reporting," Mimeo (Washington, D.C.: Georgetown University Medical Center, October 28, 1985), p. 2.
2. From an interview with Donald Berreth, CDC public relations director, April 17, 1985.
3. Remarks by HHS Secretary Margaret Heckler, International Conference on AIDS, Atlanta, Georgia, April 15, 1985.
4. Dialog's National Newspaper Index provides front page to back page indexing of the *Christian Science Monitor*, the *Wall Street Journal*, the *New York Times*, the *Washington Post*, and the *Los Angeles Times*. Each entry in the index has a short precis of the article's content. Articles retrieved from the data base in the initial period of the epidemic were categorized into five groups: (1) Personal interest: how AIDS affects lifestyle, emotional toll in patients, fears, response to the epidemic in the homosexual community; (2) Technical and educational information; (3) Announcements of new research findings, hypotheses, and speculation; (4) Policy decisions, funding decisions, and reports of how public and private institutions respond to the epidemic; and (5) Reports on the development of a test to screen blood. Whereas newspapers carried a spectrum of reports tied to events, magazines focused on personal interest stories and technical reports. Public policy journals, not surprisingly, covered the announcement of AIDS as the nation's number one health priority and discussions of the development of a blood test and a potential vaccine.

5. Reference is to Dialog's Magazine Index, which covers 435 popular magazines, and Public Affairs Information Service, which surveys over 800 English language journals and 6,000 nonserial publications for "comprehensive coverage for all issues of public policy regarding social, economic, or political problems."

6. From an interview with Lawrence Mass, December 28, 1984.

7. Ibid.

8. Dennis Altman, *AIDS in the Mind of America* (Garden City, N.Y.: Anchor Press, 1986), p. 108.

9. Jerry E. Bishop, "Epidemic," *Discover* (September 1982), pp. 35–38.

10. From conversation with Jerry Bishop, February 28, 1986.

11. See note 6 above.

12. For an interesting debate among science writers covering this story, see William Check, "AIDS/HTLV Story Raises Troublesome Issues," *Newsletter of the National Association of Science Writers*, 32 (November 3, 1984) pp. 1–6; and editorial correspondence, ibid., pp. 5–9.

13. D. D. Ho et al., "Infrequency of Isolation of HTLV-III Virus from Saliva in AIDS," *NEJM* 313 (1985) p. 1606; and S. M. Saviteer et al., "HTLV-III Exposure During Cardiopulmonary Resuscitation," ibid., pp. 1606–1607.

14. From an interview with Donald Berreth, April 8, 1985.

15. From an interview with Kenneth Sell, scientific director of NIAID, December 14, 1984.

16. From an interview with CDC Director James Mason, January 4, 1985.

17. The CDC ran a consensus conference to determine recommendation for the use of HIV antibody tests in limiting the spread of AIDS in February 1987. Recommendations formed as a result of the meeting were endorsed by the surgeon general.

18. Robert Pear, "Makers of Policy on AIDS," *New York Times*, June 12, 1987; see also Leslie Maitland Werner, "Education Chief Presses AIDS Tests," *New York Times*, May 1, 1987.

19. Christine Russell, "Balancing Check: Experts Differ on the Release of Medical News," *Newsletter of the National Association of Science Writers*, 32 (November 3, 1984), pp. 7–8: comments on an article published earlier by William Check.

20. William Check, "Public Education on AIDS: Not Only the Media's Responsibility," Hastings Center Report Special Supplement (August 1985), pp. 27–31. See also editorial correspondence in the *Newsletter of the National Association of Science Writers* of November 3, 1984.

21. "Education and Foster Care of Children Infected with Human T-Lymphotropic Virus Type III/Lymphadenopathy Associated Virus," *MMWR*, 34 (September 6, 1985), pp. 517–521.

22. James Mason used this phrase frequently in discussing the recommendations of the CDC (see ibid.) in 1985.

23. As Harry Dowling noted, in "Sydenham Hospital of Baltimore," *Journal of the History of Medicine*, 40 (January 1985), pp. 8–9: "In 1801 Baltimore's health department had been given the legal authority to isolate and hospitalize persons with communicable diseases, but not until the end of the century did it make a consistent attempt to use these measures to control infections. Although placarding of houses containing patients with contagious diseases

was begun in 1892, proper isolation was often impossible in hotels and boarding houses and especially in the crowded houses of the poor. Even in homes where there was enough space, isolation procedures were frequently defective because the decision to isolate or quarantine, and for how long, was left to the patient's own physician who was seldom an expert in such matters and furthermore was likely to be concerned more with pleasing the patient's family than with controlling the spread of the disease."

24. "Poll Indicates Majority Favor Quarantine for AIDS Victims," *New York Times*, December 20, 1985.

25. David Black, *The Plague Years* (New York: Simon and Schuster, 1986). Portions were reprinted in *Rolling Stone* (March 28, 1985).

26. Lewis H. Lapham's comment on the conference, "AIDS and the Political Right," was syndicated countrywide; see the *Washington Post*, May 10, 1985 (© 1985 by Lewis Lapham).

27. "AIDS: What Is To Be Done?" a roundtable, *Harper's* magazine, October 1985. Present were J. Leibson, M. Krim, G. Friedland, M. Silverman, A. Fettner, M. J. Sherbar, G. MacDonald, R. Bayer, S. Schultze, and E. Brandt.

28. The San Francisco AIDS Foundation, "We Can Stop AIDS," a brochure prepared by the Stop AIDS Project in partnership with the San Francisco AIDS Foundation, coordinated by Research and Decisions Incorporated, 1985.

29. Dennis Altmann, *AIDS in the Mind of America* (Garden City, N.Y.: Anchor Press, 1986), p. 43.

30. "AIDS is a Secret Soviet Weapon," *Weekly World News*, January 1, 1986.

10. Lessons for the Future

1. Institute of Medicine, "Confronting AIDS: Directions for Public Health, Health Care, and Research" (Washington, D.C.: National Academy Press, 1986).

2. Arthur M. Silverstein, *Pure Politics and Impure Science: The Swine Flu Affair* (Baltimore, Md.: Johns Hopkins University Press, 1981), p. 16.

3. P.L. 94-380.

4. Congressman Henry A. Waxman, who was the principal opponent of the swine flu bill in the House, argued that the legislation would relieve the drug and insurance companies of accountability and would set a dangerous precedent. A contrasting—and prevailing—argument in the Senate came from Senator Jacob Javits, who insisted that it was a one-year measure designed to meet an emergency and was not meant to establish a precedent. See Silverstein, *Pure Politics and Impure Science*, p. 105.

5. FDA regulates devices for use in specific circumstances. These circumstances are spelled out on the product's label. On December 6, 1985, Congressman Henry Waxman, anticipating the policy crisis looming over HTLV-III antibody testing and the insurance industry, requested clarification of the valid uses of the test. The test's label stated that it "is inappropriate to use this test as a screen for AIDS or as a screen for members of groups at increased risk for AIDS in the general population." Despite this clear statement, Waxman knew that some people planned to use the antibody test as a mandatory screen for AIDS or as a screen for members of groups at increased risk for AIDS in the general

population. Waxman therefore asked Dr. Frank Young, the commissioner of FDA, how the agency would assure that the test would not be misused.

Young responded on February 6, 1986. He cited federal statutes under which FDA can act against those who "misuse" advice, and indicated that the test's labeling would be revised to reflect broadened applications based on data obtained since initial licensing of the tests. Since the insurance industry is regulated at the state level, FDA control over the use of the ELISA test was one of the few ways by which the federal government could quickly impose national consistency in insurance issues related to AIDS. Copies of this correspondence are available from Congressman Waxman's staff.

6. The FDA approves and monitors studies by pharmaceutical manufacturers in the testing of new drugs. See, for example, W. L. Pines, "A Primer on New Drug Development," HEW Publication (FDA) #81-3021 (July 1981). Clinical investigations are awarded investigational new drug IND status through a formal process that includes spelling out the criteria by which patients can participate in clinical trials. A patient who is not enrolled in a clinical trial may on occasion be treated with a new drug under the rule for "compassionate IND." When some measure of efficacy of a new drug has been determined, but the clinical investigations have not yet been completed and the drug has not yet been licensed for sale, a patient may be able to be treated through a "therapeutic IND."

7. *Vaccine Supply and Innovation*, Publication no. IOM-85-02 (Washington, D.C.: National Academy Press, 1985); and *New Vaccine Development: Establishing Priorities, Volume I: Diseases of Importance in the United States* (Washington, D.C.: National Academy Press, 1985).

Index

Index